DEPARTMENT OF HEALTH AND SOCIAL SECURITY

010380

D0488973

On the State of
THE PUBLIC HEALTH

THE ANNUAL REPORT OF
THE CHIEF MEDICAL OFFICER OF
THE DEPARTMENT OF HEALTH AND SOCIAL SECURITY
FOR THE YEAR 1986

LONDON
HER MAJESTY'S STATIONERY OFFICE

© *Crown copyright 1987*
First published 1987

ISBN 0 11 321127 9

CONTENTS

INTRODUCTION

To the Rt. Hon. John Moore, MP
  Secretary of State for Social Services

Sir,

I have pleasure in submitting my report on the State of the Public Health during 1986.

Recently I reviewed the series of Reports produced by Chief Medical Officers since 1856 at a seminar attended by colleagues with a professional interest in the public health. The seminar concluded that the Reports have been useful as an unbiased record of topical events relating to health and as a commentary on progress and on important unsolved problems. It was suggested that in future they should contain relevant statistics not available in other publications and articles on key health issues with a national and international perspective. It is hoped to incorporate a number of these changes in the Report for 1987.

In 1986 the health scene in the UK as in many other countries was dominated by the evolution of the epidemic of infection with the virus (HIV) which underlies AIDS and the increasing public awareness of its significance. But the unique character of two other events which occurred in 1986 — different, yet each in its way of historic significance to public health — earns them mention in the opening paragraphs of this Introduction.

On the night of 26 April 1986 a massive explosion took place in a nuclear reactor at Chernobyl in the Soviet Union. Although within the UK the health effects due to the radioactive cloud proved to be minimal the explosion naturally aroused widespread public concern and tested the capacity of Governments in many countries to react to a potential nuclear emergency.

The second event was the setting up in January 1986 by the then Secretary of State of an Enquiry into 'the future of the public health function'. The terms of reference give particular emphasis to the control of communicable disease and the role of the specialty of community medicine. So far as can be determined this is the first review for at least a century. It is hoped that the Committee will report at the end of this year.

Acquired immune deficiency syndrome (AIDS) and HIV infection

During the first six months of 1987 281 cases of AIDS were reported from England to CDSC. This contrasts with 107 in the comparable period of 1986, and with the 1986 total of 298 cases. The nature of the definition of AIDS introduces an arbitrary element to the dating of a diagnosis, and there may also be delays of varying length between the diagnosis and reporting of cases. If the date of diagnosis is taken as the point of reference the epidemic curves of cases in the UK is at present exponential with a doubling time of about 10 months. A similar curve is found if deaths attributed to AIDS are plotted by date of death.

The future trend of the epidemic will depend on the number of people currently infected with the underlying virus (HIV) and the rate of incidence of new infections. Although, unfortunately there are no reliable estimates of either of these figures a total of 5,009 positive tests had been reported from England, up

1

to 30 June 1987. Almost all of these people are believed to be within the high risk groups or to have been sexual partners of persons in these groups. The high risk groups are young homosexual or bisexual males, haemophiliacs, people who have had sexual intercourse in Sub-Saharan Africa and intravenous drug abusers.

In early 1987 pilot schemes for testing ante-natal patients for HIV infection in Edinburgh and Dundee were announced. It is envisaged that this will be extended to centres in England by the end of this year. Such schemes give HIV positive women the opportunity to consider whether they wish to continue with the pregnancy, since there is an approximately even chance of their offspring being infected.

In the absence of an effective vaccine or treatment the principal means of reducing the spread of HIV is to educate the public how the virus is transmitted and how to protect themselves and others. The public information campaign which began in 1986 has continued to gather momentum and has attracted much international interest. In the first two weeks of January 1987 an AIDS leaflet was delivered to every household in the country. This was accompanied by television and cinema advertising. The broadcasting authorities gave additional 'air time' to AIDS advertising on all channels and by broadcasting 19 hours of television programmes in an 'AIDS Television Week'. In the same month a two-tier free telephone information and advice service was established to complement the campaign.

This consists of an 'AIDS telephone service' which functions 24 hours a day for 7 days a week and in which general enquiries can be answered and literature offered. Callers requiring more sensitive personal advice are referred to 'The National Advisory Service on AIDS' which operates between 10 am and 10 pm, 7 days a week. Outside these hours a back-up service is provided by 'Network, Scotland'; all calls are free. All aspects of the public education campaign, including the telephone information services, are monitored and evaluated. Results of market research reveal that the vast majority of the public now know how the virus is transmitted.

In the early part of the year I accompanied the then Secretary of State for Social Services to the USA. This trip provided considerable insight into possible strategies for caring for patients. Subsequently two conferences were held — one on the prediction of the future number of AIDS cases; the other on caring for people with AIDS. Following the latter it was announced that 14 nursing fellowships would be established to formulate ideas for nursing AIDS patients, that special training facilities for other health care professionals including community nurses, general practitioners (GPs) and hospital specialists would be provided and that a pilot scheme for an AIDS regional advice and support centre, to be jointly run by the health authority and the local authority, would be established. This centre will be in Newcastle-upon-Tyne.

AIDS research
At the end of 1986, the Medical Research Council (MRC) put forward a suggestion for a programme of directed research to develop a vaccine to prevent infection and anti-viral drugs to treat those already infected with the AIDS virus. These proposals were accepted by the Government in February 1987 and an additional £14m was allocated over the next 3 years. The programme

2

will be closely monitored by the MRC, the Department of Health (DHSS) and the Department of Education and Science (DES).

In early 1987 the Economic and Social Research Council (ESRC) outlined its plans for a programme of research to start later in the year.

The DHSS has given research into AIDS a top priority. Many health services research projects are under consideration for a 1987 start.

Zidovudine (*'Retrovir'*) was issued with a project licence by the Committee on Safety of Medicines (CSM) on 4 March 1987. Supplies are limited and its use at present is confined to the management of serious manifestations of HIV infection in patients with the AIDS syndrome or AIDS related complex (ARC).

Whooping cough

Although 1986 was an epidemic year, notified cases were considerably less than those for the equivalent epidemic years of 1978 and 1982. This fall was the result of improved immunisation but a much greater increase in uptake of pertussis vaccine is needed if future epidemics are to be avoided.

Vaccination and immunisation

The uptake of measles and whooping cough vaccine has shown some increase in recent years, but these levels together with those for diphtheria, tetanus, poliomyelitis and rubella vaccination are below the target levels of 90%.

In August 1985, and again in July 1986, the District Health Authorities were asked to designate a particular person to co-ordinate immunisation activity in each district. As the theme for World Health Day 1987 was immunisation, it was considered appropriate to hold the first meeting of these designated officers on that day, 7 April, at the London School of Hygiene and Tropical Medicine.

On 7 April 1987, it was announced that Ministers had approved a change in childhood immunisation policy to replace single antigen measles immunisation with combined measles, mumps and rubella (MMR) immunisation. This new vaccine will be introduced in the autumn of 1988 and in the meanwhile trials on the acceptance and reactivity of the vaccine are being carried out in Somerset, North Hertfordshire and Fife.

Meningitis

Britain is currently experiencing the first resurgence of meningococcal meningitis since 1976. In 1986 the notifications rose for the third succesive year to some 850 cases and a further increase is expected in 1987. As the dominant strain has been Group B for which no vaccine is at present available, it has not been possible to control the outbreak by immunisation. Although penicillin is usually effective if given in adequate doses as soon as the diagnosis is suspected there remains a significant fatality rate of about 10%. This together with the facts that it attacks principally young children and adolescents, and, as it is transmitted by undisclosed carriers, seems to strike at random account for the high degree of public concern associated with this condition.

3

The Health Education Authority

In November 1986 the then Secretary of State announced the proposed reconstitution of the Health Education Council as a special health authority. While the immediate purpose was to create a statutory body suitable to assume responsibility for the £20 million public education campaign on AIDS, this reconstitution will also enhance the importance of health promotion within the NHS. It will ensure that it is given appropriate priority in the accountability review process. The Health Education Authority (HEA) came into being on 1 April 1987, and further details of its functions and composition are given in Chapter 2.

Look after your heart!

1986 witnessed the planning of this campaign which was launched officially by the then Secretary of State in April 1987. The campaign is jointly sponsored by DHSS and the HEA, and its aim is to reduce what in international terms is in England a very high level of coronary heart disease (CHD). The first phase is largely intended to raise public awareness about the main risk factors in CHD which include smoking, dietary fat and lack of exercise and to suggest what people can do to reduce them. A fuller description of the campaign is given in the section on CHD (see page 31).

Smoking

References to the well established connections between smoking and ill health appear in various parts of the main report. However, because of its importance to the state of the public health, a special section on the subject has been included in Chapter 2 of the Report.

Although mortality from all-causes has fallen in all social classes, the decline has been least in those engaged in semi-skilled and unskilled manual work. Smoking is a major contributor to such differences, particularly with respect to coronary heart disease and lung cancer. While it would be quite wrong to express any satisfaction about the nation's smoking habits, it is encouraging that the most recent prevalence data demonstrate that the proportions of both adult men and women who smoke now show a decline in unskilled manual workers, as well as in all other socio-economic groups. There remain however large differences in smoking prevalence across society and it is important that further substantial improvements are made.

In contrast to adults, recent evidence about smoking among young people continues to give me considerable cause for concern. Although the 1986 survey on smoking among secondary school children showed that the prevalence rate for smoking in first to fifth form boys was 7% — in 1984 it had been 13% — smoking in the same group of girls remained virtually unchanged. It is particularly unsatisfactory that among fifth formers 35% of girls and 24% of boys smoked regularly or occasionally.

The effects of passive smoking — that is, the effect on the health of non-smokers of inhaling other people's tobacco smoke is now provoking increasing concern. The Independent Scientific Committee on Smoking and Health (ISCSH) issued a public statement in March 1987. The Committee confirms the association between passive smoking and the exacerbation of respiratory and cardiovascular symptoms. It also pointed out that the findings on the association between passive smoking and lung cancer were consistent with an increase in the small absolute risk of lung cancer among non-smokers — possibly of the order of 10–30%. It is likely that many non-smokers will soon expect to be able to work and to undertake leisure activities in a smoke-free environment.

Drug misuse

Drug misuse remains a major problem. Though there is some evidence from indicators of drug misuse that the availability and use of heroin may have slowed down in 1986, the widespread use of illicit amphetamine sulphate is worrying, and there is the continued threat of a rise in cocaine misuse.

HIV infection is a new major associated risk for people who inject any of these substances. Sharing of syringes, needles and other paraphernalia provides an important route for transmission of HIV and the mortality associated with HIV far exceeds that associated with drug misuse *per se*. Moreover, infected drug users may transmit the virus by sexual contact to their partners and in the case of women to the unborn child.

It is therefore even more urgent than previously to give priority to the development and expansion of local drug misuse services, so that a greater number of drug users, whether casual or dependent, may be contacted and offered advice and treatment.

Alcohol misuse

Recently additional powerful arguments have emerged in support of the need for action on alcohol as a cause of disease. It has been known many years that alcohol misuse can give rise to cirrhosis, mental illness and other disorders of the central nervous system as well as being an important factor in the causation of cancers of the upper respiratory and digestive tracts. More recently there has been growing evidence to implicate alcohol in the development of hypertension and breast cancer, both major causes of death and illness. It seems that the effects of alcohol on the development of these two conditions may be important even at relatively moderate levels of consumption in predisposed individuals. The total range of health problems in which alcohol may be a significant factor makes the drinking habits of the nation the legitimate concern of every doctor. The recent publication of special reports on alcohol by three Medical Royal Colleges and the British Psychological Society highlight the scale of the problem. A particularly welcome feature of these publications was that all four reports included a single co-ordinated series of recommendations on safe levels of alcohol consumption. The maximum levels of consumption which are thought to be safe are 21 units per week for men and 14 units per week for women. [One unit = ½ pint of ordinary beer or a standard measure of wine or spirits.]

Environmental radiation

The Department's response to the Chernobyl accident in the USSR included provision of advice to the public on the immediate implications within the United Kingdom (UK), and subsequently international collaboration to improve the guidelines on which any actions necessary in the future would be taken. The Department has also been involved in the Government's review of the UK plans for dealing with nuclear emergencies.

The Committee on Medical Aspects of Radiation in the Environment (COMARE) which was set up at the end of 1985 in response to a recommendation in the Black Advisory Group Report on the *'Investigation of the Possible Increased Incidence of Cancer in West Cumbria'* published its first report in 1986. This reassessed the findings of the Black Advisory Group in the light of additional discharge data made available by British Nuclear Fuels plc, and judged that the substance and essential conclusions of the Black Advisory Group were unchanged. COMARE also advised Government on the significance to health of exposures to radon in dwellings, and recommended that the feasibility of a study of the effects of radon exposure on inhabitants of dwellings in the UK be considered.

Cervical screening

The importance of this subject remains undiminished and the main developments in 1986 are referred to in Chapter 6. The aim of policy is to achieve a substantially greater uptake of screening — particularly among women who have never previously had a cervical smear test thereby reducing the mortality from the disease.

In February 1987 the then Secretary of State announced that call and recall for cervical cancer screening will extend to women from the age of 20 years. In April he announced the establishment of a small team, headed by Sir Roy Griffiths, which is to oversee the implementation of this Government's policies on cancer screening, in particular by ensuring that Health Authorities have viable plans to implement computer-based call and recall systems by Spring 1988.

Breast screening

Following the publication of the report of the Working Group set up to consider breast screening policy the Secretary of State also made it known that a national breast screening service was to be set up. By early 1988 each region would have one screening centre with the intention of increasing this number to 100 for the whole country by 1990.

Trials in Sweden and elsewhere have demonstrated that screening by mammograph can prolong the lives of women with breast cancer aged 50 years and over. The programme envisaged by the UK Health Ministers will require skilled and motivated multidisciplinary teams. For success to be assured it will also be necessary to persuade the majority of women of the appropriate age to avail themselves of this service.

Syringes for diabetics

About a million people suffer from diabetes in the United Kingdom and a fifth of them need regular injections of insulin to maintain their health. Prior to 1987 some were supplied with disposable syringes through the hospital service but the majority relied on re-usable syringes and needles prescribed by their GPs.

This situation was widely perceived as unsatisfactory because of possible infection through re-use of equipment, and the greater ease and comfort that would come from use of disposables. This was argued particularly strongly in respect of children. In Scotland disposables have been available on GP prescription for some time for patients up to age of 16 years.

In March 1987, the Minister for Health told the House that disposable syringes and needles would be available on GP prescription. Since diabetics are among the groups who are exempt from all prescription charges, this supply will be free, and is expected to cost up to £10 million in a full year.

Organisation and management of health services

Outcome indicators
While a great deal of information is collected about health service activity we know surprisingly little about the extent to which health services actually improve people's health. Much more needs to be done to develop indicators which enable professional staff and managers to assess the results of treatment in terms of actual benefit to patients. Decisions on priorities would be easier if we had clearer indicators of such benefits.

At present only a few measures of clinical outcome are available. A small number of the current performance indicators relate to outcome, mainly in the fields of maternity services and immunisation. Increasing interest is being shown in avoidable deaths as indicators of outcome. These measure mortality for selected diseases or conditions which can be effectively prevented or treated by district. While differences between districts must be interpreted with care, they often point to the need for local investigation of a particular problem.

A growing number of District Medical Officers are producing reports on the health of the populations of their Districts and a number of Health Authorities are adopting specific targets for health improvement as part of their longer term planning. While health services are clearly only one of many factors which influence the health of a community, the measurement of indicators of outcome of services will play an increasingly important part in determining what real benefits people derive from the NHS.

Medical equipment
A report by a working group of the Advisory Council for Applied Research and Development (ACARD) on the medical equipment industry in the UK was published in July 1986. A central theme was the importance of the NHS as an influence on the industry's shape, and the implications this has for both the home and overseas markets.

In announcing the publication of the Government's response in February 1987 the Secretary of State made clear the Government's commitment to the industry. He drew attention both to the wide-ranging programme of actions designed to develop a strong, internationally competitive health-care industry, which was announced on 15 December 1986, and to the future measures set out in the response. He emphasised the scope for British industry to assist the NHS in achieving increased efficiency, value for money and the provision of improved care, and the opportunity for building a firmer base for exports which would result if the industry could meet a higher proportion of the Service's needs.

Croham report

I welcome the attention given to developments in the field of undergraduate medical education by the Croham Report on the review of the University Grants Committee (UGC). The report contains a clear statement of the complex funding and management arrangements which apply to medical education and recommends that better co-ordination of planning and funding is needed between DHSS and DES and between Health Authorities and the Universities. The recommendations of the Report have been followed up at national level by DHSS in conjunction with DES and the UGC. Working links between the Departments have been strengthened. In March 1987 a joint note of guidance was issued by DHSS and DES to health authorities and universities with medical schools. It called for health authorities to review their resource allocation policies in the light of the needs of medical education and emphasised the need for joint planning and consultation.

The Artificial Limb Service

Brief reference was made in this Report for 1985 (p. 88) to the review of the Artificial Limb and Appliance Service (ALAC) undertaken by Professor McColl's Working Party which was published in January 1986.

The McColl Report made a series of important recommendations, which dealt with the organisation and management of the services, the nature of the limb contracts and the standard of prosthetic care. The broad thrust of the report was accepted by Ministers and already many of the recommendations have been acted upon. A recommendation of the McColl Working Party was that it would be inappropriate for these services to remain under the direct control of the DHSS. This also was accepted by the Government who therefore decided to establish an interim management board in the form of a Special Health Authority, with effect from 1 July 1987; it is known as the Disablement Services Authority and will be responsible for the whole of the artificial limb service, for wheelchair services and for the provision of appliances to war pensioners.

The Working Party also identified a need to forge stronger links with the other services for disabled people. To this end Ministers have decided that one of the major tasks of the Special Health Authority will be to prepare the way for full integration of the ALAC services into the NHS in April 1991. As part of its consideration of the longer term arrangements, the Authority will also be asked to devise any safeguards which are needed to ensure that continuity of the services is maintained, and that there is no disruption or diminution of them. The Authority itself will cease to exist after 1991 and its responsibilities will pass to regional and district health authorities.

Trends in asthma

It is my intention to select each year an aspect of the problem of disease in England which is of concern or topical interest and to subject it to detailed analysis.

The first subject in this series, bronchial asthma, which appears to have become more prevalent in recent years, is dealt with in Chapter 1 on page 24.

The Committee on Safety of Medicine (CSM)

The work of the CSM and its sub-committees during 1986 is described on page 91. A list of members during 1986 appears as Appendix A on page 141. The period of appointment for all members expired on 31 December 1986, and I would like to record my appreciation of their valuable work. In particular, Professor Sir Abraham Goldberg retired after being Chairman of the Committee since July 1980. During his 6½ years in office Professor Goldberg chaired the Committee with unfailing tact and courtesy. He will be very much missed by members and Secretariat.

Acknowledgement
I am also grateful to colleagues who have helped to prepare this Report, and to the Medical Statistics Division of the Office of Population, Censuses and Surveys.

I am, Sir
Your obedient Servant

E D Acheson
September, 1987.

1. VITAL STATISTICS

(a) Population size

The estimated resident population of England on 30 June 1986 was 47,254,000 persons, an increase of 143 thousand over that for 1985. Almost one half of the increase was due to natural change (births minus deaths) and the other half to migration. There was an increase of over 10% in the estimated number of immigrants from beyond the United Kingdom coupled with a decrease of 2% in the number of emigrants leaving England for destinations beyond the UK.

(b) Age and sex structure of the resident population

Table 1.1 shows how the size of the population in various age/sex groups has changed over recent years. There was a small increase in the number of 1–4 year olds between mid-1985 and mid-1986 which reflected aging of the 'under 1' cohort at mid-1985, this being 4% higher than the mid-1984 cohort. The number of children of school age (5–15 years) had fallen by 11% since 1981. The fall between 1985 and 1986 was the smallest for the past 5 years. The overall number of adults of working age (16–64 years for men and 16–59 years for women) continued to increase. This disguises, however, a further decrease in the working population over age 45 years. The number of people of pensionable age at mid-1986 was slightly higher than a year earlier. There were increases in all three of the pensionable age groups shown in Table 1.1; once again the largest, just under 4%, was for those aged 85 years and over. Since 1981 the number of people in the age groups of 75–84 years and 85 years and over has increased by 11% and 18% respectively. Men account for one-third of all people over retirement age, a proportion which has changed little since 1981.

Table 1.1: *Population age and sex structure 1986, and changes by age 1981–86: England*

Age	Resident population Mid-1986 Thousands			Percentage change (Persons)			
	Persons	Males	Females	1981–86	1983–84	1984–85	1985–86
Under 1	618	317	301	**3.3**	0.0	4.2	0.9
1–4	2,386	1,223	1,163	**6.8**	0.5	–0.3	1.1
5–15	6,602	3,391	3,211	**–11.4**	–2.2	–1.7	–1.4
16–29	10,464	5,312	5,153	**6.2**	1.3	1.4	0.9
30–44	9,653	4,850	4,803	**5.2**	0.1	0.1	1.5
45–64/59*	8,907	5,050	3,857	**–2.1**	0.1	–0.8	–0.1
65/60–74**	5,520	1,851	3,669	**–2.2**	–1.1	0.4	0.2
75–84	2,501	898	1,603	**11.2**	2.5	1.8	1.2
85 & over	603	142	462	**18.0**	3.2	4.1	3.8
All ages	47,254	23,034	24,220	**0.9**	0.2	0.3	0.3

* 45–64 for males, 45–59 for females
** 65–74 for males, 60–74 for females
Figures may not add due to rounding.

(c) Fertility statistics — aspects of relevance for health care

(i) Teenage conceptions
Data on conceptions to women resident in England and Wales cover pregnancies which lead to a maternity or to a legal termination under the 1967

10

Table 1.2: *Teenage conceptions: Numbers and rates, 1974 and 1984, England and Wales*

Age at conception/ Year of conception	All Conceptions	Conceptions outside marriage					Conceptions inside marriage		
		Total	*Illegitimate maternities** Sole registrations	Joint registrations	Legitimate maternities†	Abortions under the 1976 Act	Total	Maternities	Abortions under the 1976 Act
(a) *Numbers (thousands)*									
Under 16									
1974	9.4	9.3	2.7	1.0	1.1	4.5	0.0	0.0	0.0
1984	9.6	9.6	2.3	1.7	0.3	5.4	0.0	0.0	0.0
Under 20									
1974	118.2	80.1	15.7	8.4	27.5	28.5	38.1	37.0	1.1
1984	118.2	97.9	19.1	26.0	14.1	38.7	20.4	19.6	0.8
(b) *Rates per 1,000 girls*									
Under 16									
1974	8.5	8.5	2.4	0.9	1.0	4.1	0.0	0.0	0.0
1984	8.6	8.6	2.1	1.5	0.2	4.8	0.0	0.0	0.0
Under 20									
1974	69.6	47.2	9.2	4.9	16.2	16.8	22.4	21.8	0.6
1984	59.9	49.6	9.7	13.2	7.1	19.6	10.3	9.9	0.4

Notes:

Rates for the under 16 and under 20 age-groups are based upon the populations of girls aged 13–15 and 15–19 respectively.

* Illegitimate births may be registered by the mother alone (Sole) or by both mother and father (Joint).

† Conceptions outside marriage leading to legitimate births occurring less than 8 months after marriage.

Abortion Act, but do not include those leading to spontaneous abortion. In Table 1.2 the numbers and rates of girls becoming pregnant at ages under 16 years and under 20 years are compared for the years 1974 and 1984. For under-16s the conception rate per 1,000 female population aged 13–15 years was about the same in each year, although there were changes in the outcome of these pregnancies; for example, the proportion of conceptions terminated by abortion increased over the period (from 48% to 56%).

The overall teenage conception rate per 1,000 female population aged 15–19 years fell between 1974 and 1984, but legal terminations increased (rising from 25% to 33% of all conceptions to under-20s). The proportion of teenage pregnancies resulting in a birth within marriage virtually halved over the decade, whilst jointly registered illegitimate births rose steeply (from 7% to 22%).

(ii) First legitimate births to women aged 30 years and over
First births to women aged 30 years and over are of medical interest in view of the greater likelihood of obstetric problems with a first pregnancy at this age. Table 1.3 shows that there were more first births to married women of this age-group during 1986 than in 1966, when total numbers of births were near a post-war peak. Increases have mainly occurred among women aged 30–34 years, who accounted for an estimated 15% of all legitimate first births in 1986 (compared with 7% in 1966).

Table 1.3: *First legitimate births to women aged 30 years and over: 1966, 1976 and 1986, England and Wales*

Age of mother	Number of births (000s)		
	1966	1976	1986 (est.)
All ages 30 and over	29.3	24.3	39.3
30–34	20.7	19.7	30.8
35–39	7.1	3.9	7.6
40–44	1.4	0.7	0.8
45 and over	0.1	0.0	0.0

(iii) Average age of mother at first legitimate birth
Increases in the average age at which women marry and the interval between marriage and first birth serve to raise the average age at which women have children. Table 1.4 shows that between 1976 and 1986 the average age at first legitimate birth increased from 24.9 years to 26.2 years, this pattern being evident in all the social classes.

(iv) Sex ratio of births
Male live births exceeded female live births by about 5% in 1986, which was fractionally fewer than in 1976 and 1966 (about 6% more males than females born live in these two years). The ratio of male to female live births varied little for mothers of different ages.

(d) Mortality and morbidity statistics

The overall level of mortality was slightly lower in 1986 than in the previous year — with a total of 538,628 deaths (533,150 in 1985) and a crude mortality

Table 1.4: *Mean age of women at first legitimate live birth, according to social class* of husband: 1976 and 1986, England and Wales*

Social class* of husband	Mean age of woman at first legitimate birth	
	1976	1986 (est.)
All Social Classes (including 'other')	24.9	26.2
I and II	26.9	28.1
III Non-manual	25.7	26.9
III Manual	24.1	25.5
IV and V	23.1	24.2

* Definition of Registrar General's Social Classes:

Non-manual:	I	Professional occupations
	II	Intermediate occupations (including most managerial and senior administrative occupations
	IIIN	Skilled occupations (non-manual)
Manual:	IIIM	Skilled occupations (manual)
	IV	Partly-skilled occupations
	V	Unskilled occupations
Other:		Residual groups (including for example Armed Forces, students and those whose occupations were inadequately described).

rate of 11.5 per thousand population (11.7 in 1985). The weather throughout the year is an important factor influencing oscillations in numbers of deaths per week, per month, or for the total year — and there had been a more severe period of cold in 1985 than 1986. Figures 1.1 and 1.2 show the 3 main causes of deaths in males and females at different ages. The figure shows the three commonest causes of death in each of three age-groups. Infant deaths, for which the pattern of mortality is very different, are dealt with in the following sub-section. When examining figures like these, it must be remembered that the cause list utilised has a major influence on the ranking of the individual causes. Thus the contribution of cancer, which accounts for 24% of the total deaths, is minimised. The figure has been based on aggregations of causes of death to the level recommended by the World Health Organization in their Basic Tabulation List.

By the age of 35–54 years ischaemic heart disease is the commonest cause of death in males, and remains so in older age-groups. In females aged 35–54 years of age malignant neoplasm of the breast is the commonest cause of death. Other forms of malignant disease are important causes of death at this age — alimentary tract cancer in both sexes, genitourinary cancers in females and respiratory cancer in males. Although less predominant in females than in males, respiratory cancer is still the fifth commonest cause of death in women aged 55–74 years, the trends in this cancer reflecting the different smoking patterns in the sexes.

Cardiovascular disease other than ischaemic heart disease becomes an important cause of death for both males and females above the age of 55 years as do other vascular diseases. Respiratory disease is the fifth cause in males aged 55–74 years and pneumonia in females 75 years and over (and this is predominantly certificates solely mentioning bronchopneumonia and no other condition present).

Figure 1.1: *Three main causes of death at different ages (as percentage of all causes of death) males, England, 1986*

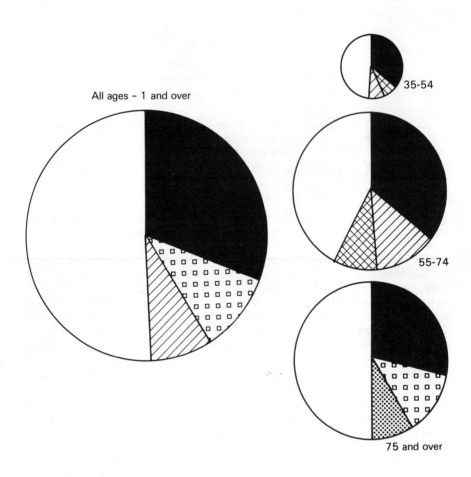

All ages – 1 and over

35-54

55-74

75 and over

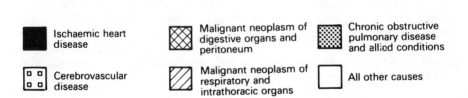

Ischaemic heart disease

Malignant neoplasm of digestive organs and peritoneum

Chronic obstructive pulmonary disease and allied conditions

Cerebrovascular disease

Malignant neoplasm of respiratory and intrathoracic organs

All other causes

Figure 1.2: *Three main causes of death at different ages (as percentage of all causes of death) females, England, 1986*

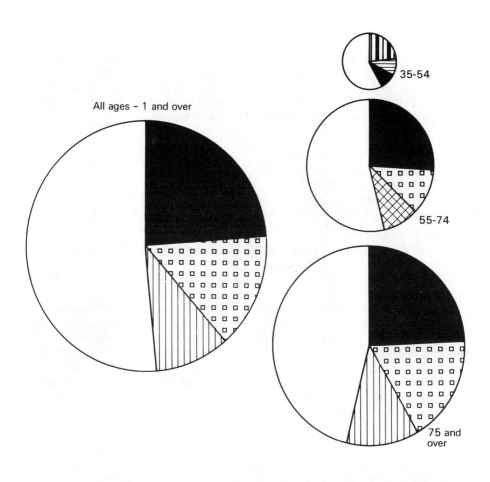

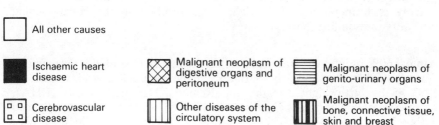

All other causes

Ischaemic heart disease

Cerebrovascular disease

Malignant neoplasm of digestive organs and peritoneum

Other diseases of the circulatory system

Malignant neoplasm of genito-urinary organs

Malignant neoplasm of bone, connective tissue, skin and breast

An important point about the Figures is that the individual circles have their size adjusted to the numbers of deaths in the age-group, so that the Figures show both the proportion of deaths at any age from a particular cause, and the relative toll from mortality in the different age-groups.

Considering the age-group 1–14 years, road vehicles accidents are the commonest cause of death in males and second commonest in females, with the females dying most frequently from congenital abnormalities. Road vehicle accident deaths rank first amongst both males and females aged 15–34 years with other causes of injury and poisoning in second place. In the third place for males and fourth for females aged 15–34 years is suicide and self-inflicted injury. This indicates the major component of deaths at these younger age-groups coming from violence of one form or another.

(i) Stillbirth and infant mortality
Survival in liveborn children is closely related to birthweight. Therefore, birthweight is an important factor in the analysis of infant mortality. Between 1983 and 1985 birthweight was stated for almost 100% of livebirths; non-statement was less than 2% for stillbirths and less than 4% for infant deaths.

Since 1975 the Office of Population Censuses and Surveys (OPCS) has been linking deaths occurring to infants with the particulars obtained at birth registration. This infant-linked file permits mortality analyses to be carried out in relation to items recorded at birth registration, including birthweight. Figure 1.3, which uses a log scale on the vertical axis, shows the survival of babies born in 1984 by birthweight groupings. Care should be taken when interpreting these data since they include stillbirths, and the birthweight distribution of stillbirths differs from that of livebirths. Although babies born dead before 28 completed weeks gestation may have birthweights higher than those of some livebirths, such births are not registerable as stillbirths under present registration practice and do not appear in the statistics. All live births are registerable irrespective of weight and gestation.

It can be seen in Figure 1.3 that at birthweights of 550g and above, the absolute number of stillbirths and infant deaths varied little between birthweight categories. However, the number of babies surviving the first year increased sharply with increasing birthweight. This resulted in the corresponding mortality rates falling sharply.

Almost 60% of infant deaths occur during the first 28 days of life (the neonatal period). Table 1.5 shows the variation in the neonatal mortality rates for 1983–85 by birthweight category and Regional Health Authority (RHA). Approximately half of all babies born in 1983–85 weighing under 1,000g died within the neonatal period. This proportion varied between 41% in North West Thames RHA and 65% in West Midlands RHA. The mortality rates fell sharply with increasing birthweight up to 3,000g. At higher weights there was little variation in rates. High mortality rates were experienced in the 'birthweight not stated' category. Some babies dying soon after birth are never weighed; it is possible that this group may have included an excess of low birthweight babies and thus have been a biased sample.

16

Figure 1.3: *Infant mortality as experienced by the 1984 England births cohort*

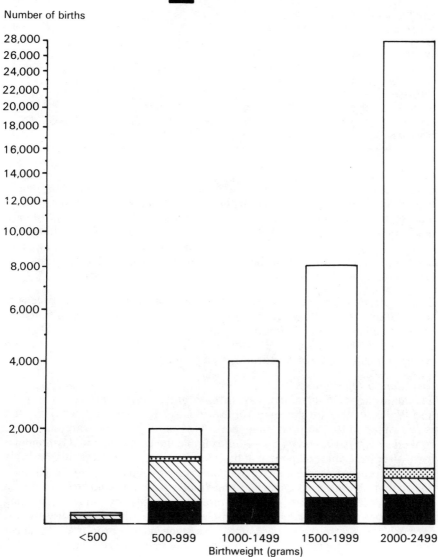

Table 1.5: *Neonatal mortality by birth weighting and RHA of residence 1983–85: Rates per 1,000 live births: England*

RHA	All weights	under 1000	1000–1499	1500–1999	2000–2499	2500–2999	3000+	Not stated
				Birth weight				
England	5.5	537.7	146.4	42.2	12.4	3.6	1.4	178.7
Northern	5.8	591.9	155.9	47.5	13.1	4.2	1.5	233.3
N Yorkshire	6.3	594.7	162.2	52.6	13.7	3.5	1.6	344.4
Trent	5.5	540.0	152.0	42.8	11.7	3.6	1.3	258.1
East Anglia	4.9	491.1	164.1	29.6	11.4	4.4	1.6	73.5
NW Thames	5.0	409.3	102.5	41.4	11.7	3.5	1.5	162.8
NE Thames	4.9	440.6	108.2	46.1	11.3	2.9	1.4	186.9
SE Thames	5.3	515.6	124.9	32.1	13.3	3.5	1.4	150.8
SW Thames	5.0	478.3	156.5	32.6	12.1	3.0	1.5	215.5
Wessex	5.2	572.7	168.9	39.0	11.2	3.4	1.6	306.9
Oxford	4.9	514.4	131.2	44.0	12.4	3.5	1.2	73.5
S Western	5.1	517.8	165.0	49.5	12.5	3.4	1.4	130.2
W Midlands	7.0	651.7	180.7	46.6	15.1	4.3	1.7	151.6
Mersey	5.2	551.1	153.8	39.5	10.4	3.5	1.2	298.9
N Western	5.6	562.2	141.2	37.3	11.1	3.8	1.3	232.9

(ii) Discharges from hospital

OPCS processes a 10% sample of discharges from non-psychiatric hospitals in England. Figures 1.4 and 1.5 show the five main causes of hospital in-patient admission (excluding maternity) at different ages and the percentage of such discharges out the total discharges by age and sex, for England in 1984. The total number of discharges varies both by age, and sex — there being more discharges amongst males in the age-groups 1–14 years and 55–74 years, but fewer discharges amongst males in the other three age-groups.

Examination of the specific causes by rank indicates both variation between the sexes, and between the different age-groups, with also appreciable differences in the stated causes and their ranks compared with the mortality data in Figures 1.1 and 1.2. This reflects the different burden of illness and hospitalisation compared with the force of mortality by age, sex and cause.

(iii) Cancer registrations

The main sites of malignant disease in males and females registered in England and Wales in 1983 are shown in Tables 1.6 and 1.7. The overall distribution is very similar to that in preceding years. There is appreciable variation in the ranked sites by age, and by sex — for example the leukaemias and lymphomas form an appreciable component at the younger ages, with a decrease from early adult life onwards; malignancies of the nervous system and related organs are also common causes of cancer in childhood compared with the elderly. In contrast the alimentary and respiratory neoplasms show increasing registrations as a proportion of all registrations in the adult and elderly groups, for both sexes. Lung cancer accounts for a much smaller proportion of cancer registrations in females than in males, whilst females show an appreciable burden from cancer of the breast and to a lesser extent cervix. A marked feature of the cervix cancer data is the relatively high proportion of neoplasms accounted for by this site in those aged 24–44 years.

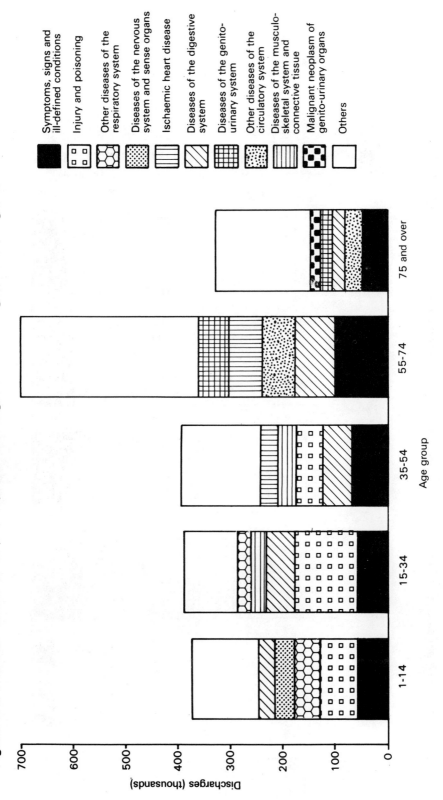

Figure 1.4: *Five main causes of hospital in-patient discharges at different ages, males, England, 1984*

Symptoms, signs and ill-defined conditions

Injury and poisoning

Other diseases of the respiratory system

Diseases of the nervous system and sense organs

Ischaemic heart disease

Diseases of the digestive system

Diseases of the genito-urinary system

Other diseases of the circulatory system

Diseases of the musculo-skeletal system and connective tissue

Malignant neoplasm of genito-urinary organs

Others

Discharges (thousands)

700
600
500
400
300
200
100
0

1-14   15-34   35-54   55-74   75 and over

Age group

Figure 1.5: *Five main causes of hospital in-patient discharges* at different ages, females, England, 1984*

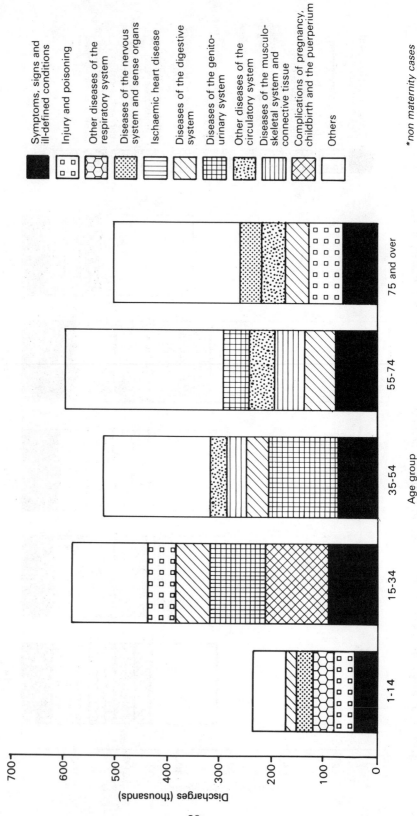

*non maternity cases

Table 1.6: *Cancer Registrations (1983) by sex, age, and site: England and Wales*

Numbers and percentages

	All ages	%	Age-group 0–4	%	5–14	%	15–24	%	25–44	%	45–64	%	65–84	%	85 and over	%
Males																
Eye, brain and other nervous system	1,795	2	61	23	73	22	75	10	286	7	802	3	490	1	8	0
Mouth and pharynx	1,827	2	3	1	6	2	21	3	124	3	722	2	865	1	86	2
Oesophagus	2,294	2	—	—	—	—	—	—	63	2	743	2	1,378	2	110	2
Lung	26,757	27	1	0	1	0	4	1	388	9	8,522	28	17,051	28	840	18
Stomach	7,060	7	—	—	1	0	1	0	128	3	1,947	7	4,640	8	343	7
Pancreas	2,881	3	—	—	—	—	—	—	80	2	855	3	1,809	3	137	3
Large intestine and rectum	11,659	12	1	0	—	—	16	2	321	8	3,411	11	7,270	12	640	14
Prostate	9,127	9	2	1	—	—	2	0	10	0	1,189	4	7,127	12	797	17
Bladder	6,683	7	1	0	1	0	9	1	149	4	1,955	7	4,254	7	314	7
Skin	12,089	12	2	1	9	3	49	6	691	17	3,947	13	6,795	11	596	13
Leukaemias and lymphomas	6,168	6	126	48	173	51	296	39	704	18	1,791	6	2,837	5	241	5
All other cancer	12,305	12	67	25	73	22	282	37	1,067	27	4,031	13	6,306	10	479	10
Total cancer	100,645	100	264	100	337	100	755	100	3,961	100	29,915	100	60,822	100	4,591	100

21

Table 1.7: *Cancer Registrations (1983) by sex, age, and site: England and Wales*

Numbers and percentages

	All ages	Age-group													
			%	0-4	%	5-14	%	15-24	%	25-44	%	45-64	%	65-84	%	85 and over	%
Females															
Eye, brain and other nervous system	1,416	1	47	22	62	24	62	10	206	3	568	2	449	1	22	0
Mouth and pharynx	1,098	1	—	—	—	—	9	2	61	1	338	1	603	1	87	1
Oesophagus	1,812	2	—	—	—	—	—	—	20	0	394	1	1,144	2	254	3
Breast	21,297	22	1	0	—	—	24	4	2,538	35	8,560	28	8,837	17	1,337	16
Lung	9,565	10	1	0	—	—	4	1	194	3	3,176	11	5,711	11	479	6
Stomach	4,493	5	—	—	—	—	3	1	66	1	714	2	3,034	6	676	8
Pancreas	2,752	3	—	—	—	—	2	0	43	1	568	2	1,807	4	332	4
Large intestine and rectum	12,453	13	3	1	—	—	12	2	303	4	2,920	10	7,623	15	1,592	19
Ovary	4,521	5	1	0	7	3	56	9	365	5	1,946	6	1,957	4	189	2
Cervix	3,875	4	—	—	—	—	38	6	1,293	18	1,405	5	1,041	2	98	1
Other uterus	3,874	4	1	0	—	—	5	1	136	2	1,742	6	1,792	4	198	2
Bladder	2,564	3	—	—	—	—	4	1	53	1	599	2	1,632	3	276	3
Skin	11,895	12	3	1	4	2	64	11	849	12	3,106	10	6,662	13	1,207	15
Leukaemias and lymphomas	5,283	5	95	45	114	44	208	35	469	7	1,267	4	2,666	5	464	6
All other cancer	10,706	11	61	29	72	28	106	18	580	8	2,757	9	6,025	12	1,105	13
Total cancer	97,604	100	213	100	259	100	597	100	7,176	100	30,060	100	50,983	100	8,316	100

(iv) Congenital malformations

The OPCS congenital malformation notification scheme only records those cases diagnosed within the first week of life. Therefore, malformations such as some heart defects, kidney conditions and sight and hearing defects, which are often not diagnosed until later in life, may not be included.

Table 1.8 shows for 1975, 1980 and 1985 the number of live and stillbirths with notified malformations to women resident in England, together with associated rates. The notification rate for live births remained steady over the period 1975 to 1985 but for stillbirths fell dramatically. However, these total rates conceal variations between individual conditions. The selected conditions given in the Table are those which have the largest number of notifications.

Over the period there was a sharp decline in notification rates for central nervous system defects. This group of malformations should be reasonably

Table 1.8: *Congenital malformation — Selected malformations, England 1975, 1980, 1985*

Malformation	Stillbirth*			Livebirth**		
	1975	1980	1985	1975	1980	1985
Any malformation						
Number	1,139	619	322	10,551	12,704	12,215
Rate	19.8	9.9	5.2	185.5	205.4	197.2
Central nervous system						
Number	929	497	114	1,159	880	571
Rate	16.2	8.0	1.8	20.4	14.2	9.2
Ear and Eye						
Number	13	22	17	340	432	673
Rate	0.2	0.4	0.3	6.0	7.0	10.9
Cleft Lip/Cleft Palate						
Number	44	49	19	767	815	758
Rate	0.8	0.8	0.3	13.5	13.2	12.2
Cardiovascular						
Number	21	16	12	574	802	775
Rate	0.4	0.3	0.2	10.1	12.9	12.5
Hypospadias/Epispadias						
Number	2	1	3	844	930	1,001
Rate	0.0	0.0	0.0	14.8	15.0	16.2
Polydactyly/Syndactyly						
Number	22	21	18	856	986	1,097
Rate	0.4	0.3	0.3	15.0	15.9	17.7
Talipes						
Number	84	43	19	2,061	2,318	1,873
Rate	1.5	0.7	0.3	36.2	37.5	30.2
Chromosomal						
Number	19	16	15	475	522	520
Rate	0.3	0.3	0.2	8.3	8.4	8.4

* Rates per 10,000 total births
** Rates per 10,000 live births

easily diagnosed at birth and therefore reported reliably. Thus the decline in notification rates probably reflects a true decrease in the incidence of these malformations. Screening and subsequent elective abortion has not been the major cause of the decline in central nervous system defect (*this Report* for 1985, p 20). The trends for some other malformations are very different to these for CNS defects.

Trends in asthma

Asthma mortality remained relatively stable from the start of the twentieth century until the beginning of the 1960s when a sharp increase was noted in several countries. Younger age-groups were particularly affected, and in the United Kingdom mortality from asthma in persons aged 5 to 34 years trebled between 1959 and 1966. Greenberg[1] suggested there was a hazard from excess use of aerosol bronchodilators for treatment of asthma, and in 1967 the Committee on Safety of Drugs issued a warning on their use to all doctors in England and Wales. Inman and Adelstein[2] demonstrated that following this both aerosol sales and deaths from asthma declined. However over-use of bronchodilators was never proven as the cause of the increased mortality, and it is now believed that excessive aerosol usage may simply reflect failure of this therapy to resolve severe attacks in some cases. Other causes have been proposed, such as inadequate therapy with systemic steroids early in the course of exacerbations of asthma.

Recently there have been reports of pronounced increases in asthma mortality in New Zealand[3] and to a lesser extent the USA[4]. Although a large increase in sales of several different drugs used in asthma treatment occurred during 1975–1981 in New Zealand, there is little evidence that the mortality trends are a direct reflection of drug toxicity[5]. Mortality trends in England and Wales have been examined by several investigators[6,7]. Khot and Burn[6] studied the mortality of children and young adults aged 5–34 years in England and Wales during 1960–82. They concluded that superimposed on seasonal variation, there had been a minimal upward drift in asthma mortality in the most recent years.

Burney[7] performed a more sophisticated analysis of asthma deaths up to the age of 64 years. This took account of a major change in coding rules relating to asthma introduced in the 9th International Classification of Diseases (ICD) in 1979, which resulted in an artefactual 28% increase in deaths attributed to asthma[8]. Burney reported a statistically significant annual mortality increase of nearly 5% a year in the age-group 5–34 years between 1974 and 1984. However interpretation of short-term trends is difficult as they reflect a wide range of inter-related factors such as changes in disease incidence, use of diagnostic aids, diagnostic fashion, disease natural history and effectiveness of treatment, as well as changes in death certification practice of doctors.

Figures 1.6 and 1.7 show selected age-specific trends for asthma mortality between 1951 and 1985. At younger ages numbers of deaths are small resulting in marked oscillations. Examination of long-term trends is complicated, particularly at older ages, by changes which have occurred in the ICD revisions. Nevertheless the figures do not suggest a recent major increase in deaths similar to that which occurred in the early 1960s. Data have also been examined according to year of birth, but this gives no clear indication of the occurrence of a cohort phenomenon.

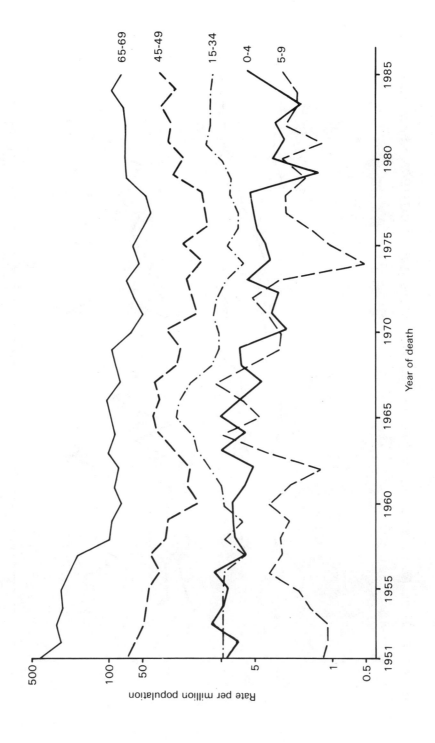

Figure 1.6: Deaths from asthma: year of death, males, England and Wales 1951-1985. Rate per million population.

25

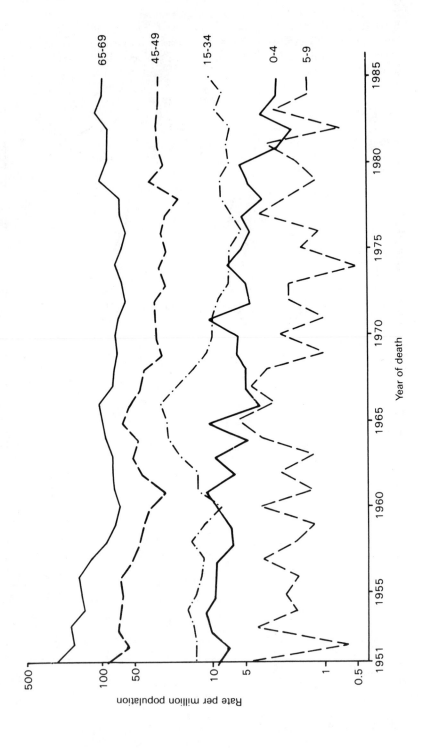

Figure 1.7: *Deaths from asthma: year of death, females, England and Wales 1951-1985. Rate per million population.*

There is a widespread belief that most deaths from asthma should be preventable[9]. However in England and Wales in 1985, 1,972 people died from the disease. About 50% of such deaths occurred in people aged under 65 years. Charlton et al[10] examined mortality ratios standardised for age for various 'avoidable' causes of death, and found an eightfold variation in asthma mortality amongst area health authorities in England and Wales. (Standardised mortality ratios in persons aged 5–49 years ranged 31–249). Several studies have been performed into the circumstances surrounding asthma deaths and all have reached largely similar conclusions concerning areas where improvement in care needs to be offered. The British Thoracic Association carried out a confidental enquiry into adult deaths from asthma occurring in 1979. They suggested that 77 out of 90 patients (86%) had potentially preventable factors contributing to the deaths. They stressed the need for closer overall supervision of asthmatics including careful attention to patient education, earlier and more intensive treatment and pre-arranged immediate admission to hospital for asthma emergencies.

Death from asthma is relatively rare, and it is important to examine data relating to morbidity as well as mortality. The data for hospital discharge statistics have been abstracted for five age-groups, using relatively broad categories at older ages. The data shown in the Figures 1.8 and 1.9 indicate the age-specific trends over the period 1957–84. The immediate point identifiable from both graphs is a relatively steady increase in the discharge rate in the younger two age-groups (this is plotted on a log scale and the slopes for each of the curves can be compared). For the ages 15–44 years, 45–64 years, and 65+ there has been relatively little change in the statistics over the past 20 years, though the young adults show some increase. In the two youngest groups the rise is particularly from the 1970s and is more marked in the youngest age-group, who now have a discharge rate much higher than at any other age. These data have also been plotted by year of birth. There was no clear indication that this is a cohort phenomenon, though there are problems in interpreting the data because of broad age-groups used, and the difficulty in identifying overlapping time periods for the different cohorts.

Anderson et al[12] examined in-patient care of acute childhood asthmatics in the South West Thames region in 1970–78. They reported that the steady increase in the number of admissions in this period was partly due to an increase in re-admission rate, and that there had been an appreciable increase in self-referrals. These patients had less severe asthma on admission and a higher re-admission rate than patients referred by their general practitioners (GPs). Khot et al[13] investigating the national increase in asthma admissions in children, considered the rise due to either an increase in the incidence of acute childhood asthma or a swing away from primary to hospital care. Implementation of 'open-door' schemes as proposed by Crompton et al[14] would lead to this pattern of earlier hospital referral, and increased self-referral and re-admission.

Many attacks of asthma are not of sufficient severity to require hospital admission. Fleming and Crombie[15] used data from the three national morbidity surveys performed in England and Wales in 1955–6, 1970–1 and 1981–2 to study asthma trends in general practice. The annual period prevalence of asthma reported in the first study was lower than that in either of the two subsequent studies. Detailed data were available from the later studies

27

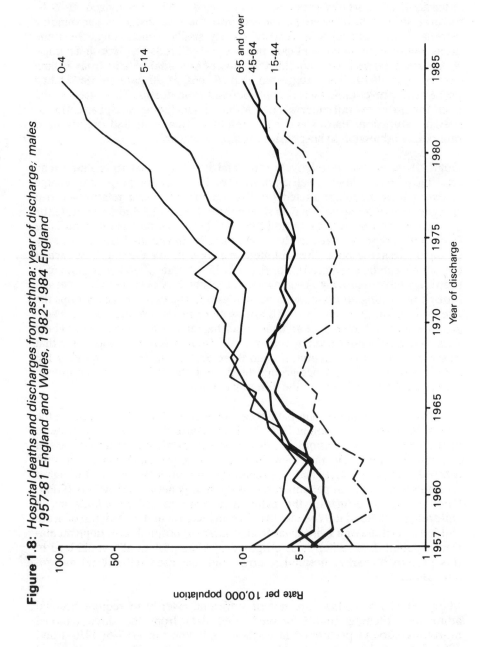

Figure 1.8: Hospital deaths and discharges from asthma: year of discharge, males 1957-81 England and Wales, 1982-1984 England

0-4

5-14

65 and over
45-64
15-44

Rate per 10,000 population

1957   1960   1965   1970   1975   1980   1985

Year of discharge

28

Figure 1.9: *Hospital deaths and discharges from asthma: year of discharge, females, 1957-81 England and Wales, 1982-1984 England*

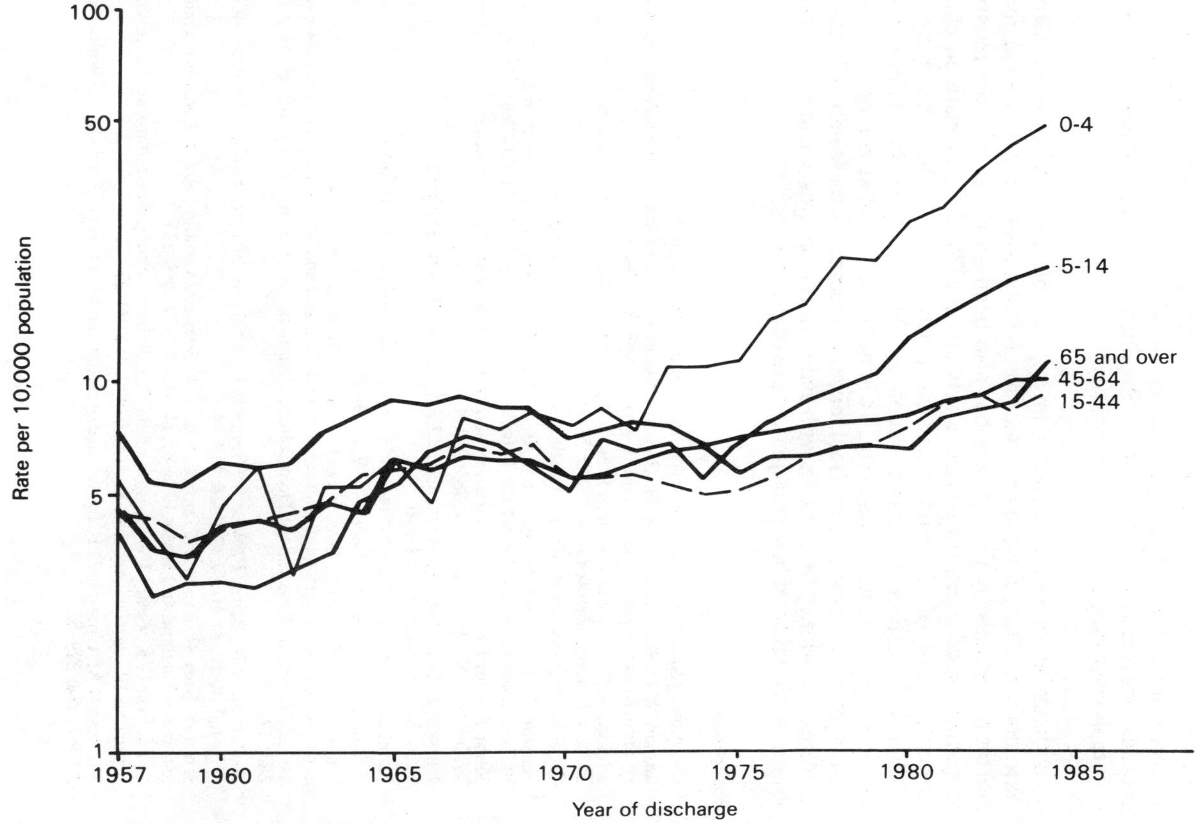

0-4

5-14

65 and over
45-64
15-44

Rate per 10,000 population

100
50
10
5
1

1957
1960
1965
1970
1975
1980
1985

Year of discharge

by age and sex and demonstrated a rise in prevalence of asthma (approximately two-fold in boys) between 1970 and 1981 with some increase seen in all age-groups and in both sexes. Examination of further statistics on consultation patterns revealed that although there was an appreciable rise in the rate of patients consulting with asthma, the number of episodes and consultations for asthma per person consulting decreased between the two surveys in both men and women. This may indicate increased diagnosis of milder cases or improved management by the GPs. Referrals to hospital represented only a very small proportion of the total of patients consulting for asthma, but did show an increase between 1970 and 1981, the increase being virtually confined to referrals requiring emergency admission.

In conclusion, there is evidence of an appreciable increase in the prevalence of patients consulting their practitioner for asthma, associated with an increase in hospital referrals by GPs. There has also been an increase in the number of in-patient spells occurring particularly since 1970 and especially in children under the age of 15 years. Over the period 1951–85 there has been some reduction in asthma mortality mainly at older ages, but in recent years this decline has become inconsistent. It is not clear to what extent these trends represent a true rise in asthma incidence, a change in disease natural history, an increased tendency for patients with asthmatic symptoms to consult their GP or an increasing role of hospitals in the care of asthmatics.

References

[1] Greenberg M J. Isoprenaline in myocardial failure. *Lancet* 1975; **ii:** 442–3.
[2] Inman W H W, Adelstein A M. Rise and fall of asthma mortality in England and Wales in relation to use of pressurised aerosols. *Lancet* 1969; **2:** 279–85.
[3] Jackson R T, Beaglehole R, Rea H H, Sutherland D C. Mortality from asthma: a new epidemic in New Zealand. *Br Med J* 1982; **285:** 771–4.
[4] Sly R M. Increases in deaths from asthma. *Ann Allergy* 1984; **53:** 20–5.
[5] Keating G, Mitchell E A, Jackson R, Beaglehole R, Rea H. Trends in sales of drugs for asthma in New Zealand, Australia and the United Kingdom, 1975–81. *Br Med J* 1984; **289:** 348–51.
[6] Khot A, Burn E. Seasonal variation and time trends of deaths from asthma in England and Wales 1960–82. *Br Med J* 1984; **289:** 233–4.
[7] Burney P G J. Asthma mortality in England and Wales: evidence for a further increase, 1974–84. *Lancet* 1986; **2:** 333–6.
[8] Lambert, P M. Oral theophylline and fatal asthma. *Lancet* 1981; **ii:** 200–1.
[9] Editorial. Fatal asthma. *Lancet* 1979; **2:** 337–8.
[10] Charlton, J T H, Hartley R M, Silver R, Holland W W. Geographical variation in mortality from conditions amenable to medical intervention in England and Wales. *Lancet* 1983; **i:** 691–96.
[11] British Thoracic Association: Deaths from asthma in two regions of England. *Br Med J* 1982; **285:** 1251–5.
[12] Anderson H R, Bailey P, West S. Trends in hospital care of acute childhood asthma 1970–8: a regional study. *Br Med J* 1980; **28:** 1191–4.
[13] Khot A, Burn R, Evans N, Lenny C, Lenny W. Seasonal variation and time trends in childhood asthma in England and Wales 1975–81. *Br Med J* 1984; **289:** 235–7.
[14] Crompton G K, Grant I W B, Bloomfield P. Edinburgh emergency asthma admission service: report on 10 years' experience. *Br Med J* 1979; **2:** 1199–201.
[15] Fleming D M, Crombie D L. Prevelance of asthma and hay fever in England and Wales. *Br Med J* 1987; **294:** 279–83.

2. PREVENTION

(a) Health Education Authority

Background
On 21 November 1986, the Secretary of State announced that he had decided to reconstitute the Health Education Council (HEC) as a special health authority. The main purpose was to create a statutory body suitable to assume responsibility for the £20 million public education campaign on AIDS, in addition to the normal health education programmes.

The relevant Order and Regulations came into effect on 3 February 1987, and the new Authority — the Health Education Authority — took over from the Council on 1 April 1987. The Chairman is Sir Brian Bailey, who has been Chairman of the Council since 1983.

Functions of the Authority
The Authority's functions are:

(a)   advising the Secretary of State for Social Services on matters relating to health education;

(b)   undertaking health education activity;

(c)   for that purpose, planning and carrying out national and regional or local programmes in co-operation with other authorities and organisations;

(d)   sponsoring research and evaluation in relation to health education;

(e)   assisting the provision of appropriate training in health education;

(f)   preparing, publishing or distributing material relevant to health education; and

(g)   providing a national centre of information and advice on health education.

It is hoped that the reconstitution of the HEC as a special health authority will give added emphasis both within the NHS and generally to the importance of health promotion within the NHS. As an integral part of the health service the Authority will participate with other health authorities in planning health service policies and priorities, and it is hoped that its involvement in the accountability service process will improve the effectiveness and efficiency of its programmes.

(b) Coronary heart disease

Coronary heart disease (CHD) is the leading cause of death among adults of both sexes in England and Wales (Table 2.1). In spite of some indication of a downward turn in the trend of mortality the countries of the UK are poorly situated in the ranking order in terms of deaths from this cause.

Steadily accumulating evidence from many countries, summarised in a series of WHO publications, the most recent in 1986[1], makes it clear that reduction in the level of risk factors known to affect the level of mortality from CHD can reduce the incidence of the disease. In England success will require changes on the part of many people in behaviour and personal lifestyle with regard to such matters as smoking, diet and exercise.

Table 2.1: *Principal causes of death, England and Wales, 1985*

| | Number | | Percentage | |
	Males	Females	Males	Females
Coronary heart disease	91,626	71,478	31.34	23.95
Cancer	74,324	67,294	25.42	22.55
Respiratory disease	34,065	30,542	11.65	10.24
Cerebrovascular disease	27,590	45,629	9.44	15.29
All other causes	64,722	83,464	22.14	27.97
Total deaths	292,327	298,407	100.00	100.00

Source: Office of Population Censuses and Surveys.

In 1984 *this Report* devoted a section to Diet and Cardiovascular Disease (p. 63) and reviewed the report of the COMA panel, published that year[2], which recommended changes in the national diet in the direction of reduced total fat intake and a reduced proportion of saturated fats. In 1985 an important publication[3] reported interim results from the Regional Heart Study. This survey looked at risk factors for major CHD (acute myocardial infarction or sudden death) in a study of 7,735 men aged 40 to 55 years drawn from general practices in 24 British towns. The report showed that after a mean follow-up of 4.2 years there had been 202 cases of major CHD. Serum total cholesterol, systolic and diastolic blood pressure, cigarette smoking and body mass index were all associated with an increased risk of CHD.

An important outcome of the Regional Heart Study has been the development of a method of estimating a 'risk score' which can be used in the conditions of general practice in order to identify men at high risk. In November 1986 the Department sponsored a conference at the Royal College of General Practitioners chaired by the Chairman of Council at which this work was presented together with other studies concerned with the prevention of CHD in general practice. This was to be followed up in the Spring of 1987 with a major one-day multidisciplinary scientific conference on progress in the prevention of CHD held at the Royal College of Physicians in London.

For some years the Government had been concerned about the high incidence of coronary disease in the UK in relation to that in some other countries. The prevalence of CHD is highest amongst the lower socio-economic groups and these have proved the hardest to reach effectively with health education messages. The Welsh Heart Programme is a major national demonstration project to promote good health in the Welsh population. It is particularly concerned with reducing the risks of cardiovascular disease throughout the whole population of the Principality by encouraging non-smoking, healthy nutrition, regular exercise, control of hypertension and first-aid for heart attacks. The programme, which is jointly funded by the Health Education Authority (HEA) and the Welsh Office, was publicly launched on 1 March 1985 for a five-year period under the title *'Heartbeat Wales'* and has already attracted considerable lay, professional, political and media interest, both at home and abroad.

In 1985 Ministers approved proposals for an extension of the CHD prevention programme in England involving:

(a)   increased emphasis on the harmful effects of smoking with particular emphasis on young people;

(b)   action on diet;

(c)   a review of preventive health arrangements by Regional Health Authorities; and

(d)   increased support for relevant voluntary bodies.

In particular an initiative was planned making extensive use of the media and with an explicitly popular image. The campaign was launched in April 1987 under the title *'Look after your Heart!'*. It is being funded and undertaken jointly by DHSS and the HEA. It will concentrate on direct communication with the public both nationally and locally, supported by parallel efforts directed at the medical profession and the NHS. It will also exploit the knowledge gained from the Welsh heart programme *'Heartbeat Wales'*. The immediate aim of the project is to increase public awareness and support for healthy lifestyles as a goal for all with particular emphasis on bringing about a decline in smoking, the adoption of healthier eating habits and of increased levels of exercise participation.

What is being sought over the longer term is a downward trend in the worryingly high incidence of CHD in England. Such an outcome will require a concerted national effort from many other statutory and voluntary bodies and the media in addition to Government, the NHS and the HEA. Improvement in other conditions related to the above risk factors, eg smoking related diseases and stroke, is also seen as an aim.

By contrast with North America, professional opinion in Britain has adopted a generally cautious approach to the possibility of preventing CHD by the population as a whole adopting lifestyle changes. However, following the Canterbury Conference of 1983, (*this Report* for 1983, p. 123), a National Co-ordinating Committee was set up under the auspices of the Royal College of Physicians to bring together the many professional and voluntary bodies with a contribution to make to the prevention of CHD. The unequivocal support of this Committee for a range of measures, including an expanded programme of health education, has been a significant factor in helping to generate a climate of opinion favourable to more positive action. Whether coincidentally or not, the year saw the publication in the national press of numerous articles on the subject of CHD, and several programmes devoted to 'healthy living' themes. The specific question of prevention of heart disease appeared on television (eg *'Don't Break your Heart'*). The public's response to this media activity appears to be favourable and positive although it will, of course, be a number of years before the outcome can be evaluated.

References

[1] World Health Organization. Expert Committee on Community Prevention Control of Cardiovascular Disease. *Community prevention control of cardiovascular disease*. Geneva: World Health Organization, 1986. (WHO technical report series; 732).

[2] Panel on Diet in Relation to Cardiovascular Disease. Department of Health and Social Security. Committee on Medical Aspects of Food Policy. *Diet and Cardiovascular disease: report of the Panel on Diet in relation to cardiovascular disease.* London: HMSO, 1984. (Report on Health and Social Subjects; 28).

[3] Shaper A G, Pocock S J, Walker M, *et al.* Risk factors for ischaemic heart disease: The prospective phase of the British Regional Heart Study. *J Epidemiol Commun Health* 1985; **39:** 197–209.

(c) Smoking and health

Smoking prevalence
Prevalence of cigarette smoking in Great Britain fell from 46% in 1972 to 34% in 1984. Among men prevalence fell from 52% in 1972 to 36% in 1984, a decline of almost one-third. Among women the proportion who smoked cigarettes fell from 41% to 32% over the same period, a fall of about one-fifth. During this period, therefore, not only was there a substantial decline in the prevalence of smoking in both sexes but the gap between the sexes narrowed. Although the peak in the annual numbers of deaths from lung cancer occurring among men in England and Wales has passed, the toll among women continues to rise and now approaches about 10,000 deaths per year. This feature reflects the later spread of cigarette smoking among women.

Smoking among children
In terms of achieving an improvement in personal health it is never too late to stop smoking. Nevertheless, the most effective public health measures are those which prevent young people taking up the habit in the first place. As indicated above efforts to discourage the habit, some sponsored or supported by the Government, have achieved a measure of success in reducing the prevalence of smoking among adults. But the take-up of smoking among young people is still worryingly high. A 1986 OPCS survey, as yet unpublished, found that 10% of first to fifth formers were 'regular smokers'. This is an improvement on the 1984 position when the comparable figure was 13%[1]. The latest survey showed a prevalence rate for smoking in first to fifth form boys of 7% but among girls in the same group the rate remained virtually unchanged at 12%.

On past evidence many teenage smokers will persist in the habit as adults and thus run the risk of developing serious, possibly fatal, smoking-related diseases in adult life. Among women the position looks particularly serious.

Teenage anti-smoking campaign
In December 1985 the Department launched a £1 million pilot media campaign aimed at discouraging teenagers from smoking. The campaign which was carefully designed to appeal to the adolescent age-group, was carried out in two TV regions, using television and the cinema. An evaluation report is being prepared and the advisability of a national campaign will be considered in the light of the findings.

Protection of Children (Tobacco) Act 1986
This Act began as the Tobacco Products (Sales Restriction) Bill, a Private Member's Bill introduced by Mr John Home Robertson, MP. The proposals were widely welcomed, and the Government gave the measure its full support. The Act makes it illegal to sell any tobacco product to children aged under 16 years irrespective of the person for whose use the product is intended. By defining tobacco to include tobacco products intended for oral or nasal use, the Act brings Skoal Bandits and similar products within its scope. With all tobacco products on the same footing as cigarettes the law is simplified, clarified and made easier to enforce. There will no longer be room for doubt as to whether a vendor is acting illegally in knowingly selling a tobacco product to someone

under the age of 16 years. All concerned with enforcing these provisions, the aim of which is to protect children, are likely to welcome the clarification.

Voluntary agreements with the tobacco industry
The Government's policy for the limitation and control of advertising and sales promotion of cigarettes continues to rely on voluntary agreements freely negotiated and entered into by the tobacco industry. A new voluntary agreement to govern the advertising and promotion of tobacco products, and health warnings, came into effect on 1 April 1986 and will run until 31 October 1989. Its main provisions are:

(a)   Advertising of cigarettes in cinemas to cease;

(b)   In place of the present health warning for cigarettes and hand-rolling tobacco there will be 6 new messages that will be given roughly equal exposure on packs, posters and press advertisements. The wording of new warnings are:

—   Smoking Can Cause Fatal Diseases
—   Smoking Can Cause Heart Disease
—   Smoking When Pregnant Can Injure your Baby and Cause Premature Birth
—   Stopping Smoking Reduces the Risk of Serious Diseases
—   Smoking Can Cause Lung Cancer, Bronchitis and Other Chest Diseases
—   More than 30,000 People Die Each Year in the UK from Lung Cancer.

The new warnings are ascribed to the Health Departments' Chief Medical Officers;

(c)   The space provided for the health warning and tar ratings on posters and press advertisements will be increased;

(d)   The industry will spend £1 million each year for the duration of the agreement on a campaign with the retail trade, supported by media advertising and direct mail, against illegal sale of cigarettes to children under the age of 16 years;

(e)   New rules to prevent cigarette posters being positioned close to schools; and

(f)   No cigarette advertisements will appear in magazines with a female readership of over 100,000, where one-third or more of those readers are aged between 15 and 24 years.

The agreement represents an advance on the previous one. Not only are the public in general provided with clearer messages about the specific dangers to health from smoking, but steps are to be taken to protect particularly vulnerable groups in the population such as children, young people and young women in the early child-bearing years.

Included in the agreements was a provision for setting up a joint committee, including representatives of government and the tobacco industry, under an independent Chairman to monitor compliance not only with this agreement but also with the separate agreement, negotiated later in the year and concluded in January 1987, on sports sponsorship by tobacco manufacturers. In November 1986, Sir Peter Lazarus, formerly Permanent Secretary at the Department of Transport, was appointed Chairman of the new committee which will be funded equally by the DHSS and the industry and will have a maximum of 14 members representing Government and the tobacco industry in equal numbers. It will meet at least 4 times a year. The Chairman is required to report annually to Ministers and the industry.

The Committee will fulfil its function in 2 main ways. It will consider complaints about breaches of the agreements sent to Government Departments or received direct, and make recommendations to resolve disputes. It will also appoint consultants to investigate aspects of the operation of the agreement and will make any necessary recommendations to the industry or Government arising from consideration of the consultant's report.

Passive smoking
There has been increasing concern over the effects of environmental tobacco smoke (so called 'passive smoking') on the health of non-smokers and during the year findings from a wide range of investigations have been published together with reviews by a number of organisations in the UK, USA and elsewhere[2,3,4,5]. In considering the additional information that has become available the ISCSH noted in an interim statement[6] that associations between passive smoking and exacerbation of respiratory and cardiovascular symptoms have been confirmed, while in respect of links with lung cancer there have been both positive and negative results. It was concluded that while none of the studies could on its own be accepted as unequivocal, the findings overall were consistent with a small increase in the risk of lung cancer among non-smokers from exposure to environmental tobacco smoke, possibly between 10% and 30%.

The vast majority of the 36,000 lung cancer deaths occurring annually in England and Wales are attributable to 'active' smoking, but the passive smoking risk could account for several hundred of the lung cancer cases arising annually in non-smokers. Attention was drawn in the statement not only to the home environment as an important source of tobacco smoke exposure, but also to the work and indoor leisure environments. The Committee noted that segregation was likely to provide better protection for non-smokers than increased ventilation. The publicity accorded to this topic through the HEC and otherwise is intended to encourage action on a voluntary basis for the provision of smoke-free environments for the two-thirds of the population who do not smoke, and the newly-formed HEA has been asked to take account of the ISCSH statement when considering educational work concerning the dangers of smoking.

References

[1] Dobbs Joy, Marsh A. *Smoking among secondary school children in 1984: an enquiry carried out for the Department of Health and Social Security, the Welsh Office and the Scottish Home and Health Department.* London: HMSO, 1985.

[2] Wald N J, Nanchahal K, Thompson S G, Cuckle H S. Does breathing other people's tobacco smoke cause lung cancer? *Br Med J* 1986, **293:** 1217–22.

[3] United States. Department of Health and Human Services. *The Health consequences of involuntary smoking: a report of the surgeon general: 1986.* Rockville (Maryland 20857): United States Department of Health and Human Services, Office on Smoking and Health, 1986.

4 Board on Environmental Studies and Toxicology. Committee on Passive Smoking National Research Council (US). Environmental tobacco smoke: measuring exposures and assessing health effects. Washington DC: National Academy Press, 1986.

5 National Health and Medical Research Council. *Report of Working Party on effects of passive smoking on health.* Canberra: AGPS, 1986.

6 Independent Scientific Committee on Smoking and Health. Interim statement on passive smoking. *Hansard* 1987, March 13: 169 (Col 2)–170 (Col 1). (Written answer).

(d) Nutrition

Cardiovascular disease

The Panel on Diet and Cardiovascular Disease of the Committee on Medical Aspects of Food Policy (COMA) reported in 1984 (see reference[2] page 34). Since that time dissemination of its recommendations has led to growing public interest in the subject. Unprecedented media attention has fostered some less moderate views than those put forward by the Panel, and the Department has acted to provide a reliable source of information by collaborating with other Government Departments (eg DES) and the HEC (now HEA) to deliver the real message. Furthermore, to take account of rapidly increasing knowledge in this field, COMA has established an Ongoing Review Panel on Diet and Cardiovascular Disease which will provide up-to-date guidance on this matter as and when necessary.

Dietary sugars

International interest in the role of sugars in the diet has continued. The US Food and Drug Administration's Task Force on Sugars reported in 1986. This has been a major contribution to the discussion, but since it inevitably dealt with matters from a US perspective, the Department felt that it was necessary to look at the issues from the UK point of view. Accordingly COMA has agreed to set up a Panel to Examine the Role of Dietary Sugars in Human Disease, with particular emphasis on the UK aspects of the problem.

Children

High priority has continued to be given to the nutritional surveillance of children. One area of concern noted by the COMA Panel on Diet and Cardiovascular Disease was that of overweight in childhood. Furthermore, the change in legislation in 1980, which removed the requirement on local authorities to provide school meals to given nutritional standards, provided the stimulus for COMA to commission a Dietary Survey of Schoolchildren in Great Britain. In 1986 a preliminary report of this survey was published; 3,285 children aged between 10 and 11, and 14 and 15 years, who all prepared 7-day weighed dietary records, and underwent height and weight measurement, were examined in the survey. The main findings were in general reassuring — there was little evidence of nutritional deficiencies, although older girls tended to have rather lower intakes of iron and some other nutrients than the rest of the population. The proportion of energy which was derived from fat, however, was 39–45% — much higher than the 35% level recommended by the COMA Panel. It was concluded that further education of this sub-group of the population in nutritional matters was needed to bring about beneficial changes in their eating habits.

Adults

Up to now, the dietary intakes of members of the adult population have been derived from estimates of foods entering households. These were obtained by the National Food Survey, carried out by the Ministry of Agriculture, Fisheries and Food (MAFF). Direct measurements of dietary habits have been limited to smaller non-representative studies. In 1986, therefore, the Department in conjunction with MAFF and OPCS, set up a Dietary and Nutritional Survey of a nationally representative sample of 2,000 adults in Great Britain. Together with a 7-day weighed dietary record, heights and weights and other anthropometric measurements are being taken to give a better indication of body fatness, as well as haematological and biochemical measures of nutritional status from those respondents willing to provide a blood specimen. In addition a 24 hour urine sample is being collected and blood pressure measured. It is hoped that this unique in-depth survey of a representative sample of the adult population will provide valuable baseline demographic information, and allow many interrelationships between diet and 'risk factors' for disease to be elucidated. The question of instituting a follow-up study of the sample is being considered.

(e) Drug misuse

Prevention remains a key element in the Government's overall strategy directed to drug misuse. The momentum of the prevention campaign has been maintained during the year. The mass media campaign, specifically targetted at young people, emphasised the adverse social consequences arising from drug misuse including those which bear upon personal relationships. Towards the end of the year, in the context of AIDS, the new dangers of injected drugs were highlighted. Evaluation so far suggests that the breakdown of social relationships has been a particularly effective message in reinforcing young people's attitudes away from drug use.

An educational video package, *'Double Take'*, for use with 13–15 year olds was made available to all secondary schools in 1986. An evaluation of its use and effectiveness is under way.

Following on the £17.5 million made available from central funds in 1984 to stimulate the development of local services for drug misuse, an additional £5 million was allocated to Regional Health Authorities (RHAs) in 1986/87 to develop these services. The Department is monitoring the use of these resources.

In addition to clinial services, it is pleasing to note the implementation of a wide range of advice and counselling centres, telephone helplines, and projects providing recreational facilities and work experience for young people at risk. These are all important preventive developments.

A Drug Advisory Service, under the auspices of the Health Advisory Service (HAS) has been set up to provide a source of advice and expertise to individual District Health Authorities (DHAs). The Drug Advisory Teams are unique in including a representative from the voluntary sector, who have long experience in early intervention and rehabilitation in the drug field. Five visits took place in 1986. It is encouraging that requests for visits have been received from other DHAs.

In addition, a major research project to review and assess the impact of the central funding initiative, and to evaluate the effectiveness of the projects began in October 1986.

(f) Alcohol misuse

Alcohol misuse now costs the nation more than £1800 million every year[1].

Financial costs are only one aspect of the burden of alcohol-related harm but give some idea of the magnitude of the problem. It is therefore a matter of great concern that the annual consumption of alcohol per head of population rose again in 1985 to 9.3 litres and that indicators of alcohol-related harm are generally following the same upward trend.

This concern is reflected in a number of events which combined to focus attention more sharply on alcohol during 1986 and 1987.

Special reports on alcohol

The Royal College of Psychiatrists, Royal College of General Practitioners, Royal College of Physicians and the British Psychological Society each published a special report on alcohol.[2,3,4,5] The Reports emphasise the potentially serious consequences of the rising trend in alcohol consumption and call for preventive action at both national and local levels. Of particular importance is the recent appreciation of alcohol consumption as a major and potentially reversible cause of hypertension and a possible predisposing factor towards breast cancer in women. The professional bodies behind these and other reports co-ordinated their recommendations on safe levels of alcohol consumption at around 21 units per week for men and 14 units per week for women*. A British Medical Association Report on Young People and Alcohol[6] highlighted the special risks to the young from episodic consumption of large quantities of alcohol. Road accidents, many of them alcohol-related are a major cause of death among young people. The Department supported an international symposium on *'Young Drivers Alcohol and Drug Impairment'* organised in Amsterdam by the International Drivers' Behaviour Research Association.

The OPCS published the findings of its Review of Adolescent Drinking, commissioned by the Department[7]. The Report suggested that, while the most young drinkers consume only modest quantities, for a worrying minority, drinking to excess is an established habit. Underage drinking in pubs was reported to be a common occurrence.

Licensing laws

The Home Office announced Government support in principle for some relaxation of the present Licensing laws in England and Wales. The Home Secretary recognised the public health implication of any proposed increase in availability of alcohol and emphasised the importance of maintaining adequate and effective controls of licensed outlets.

Centrally funded research

The Department published a Review of Alcohol Detoxification Services[8] commissioned by the Homelessness and Addictions Research Liaison Group.

Conferences

Lack of awareness among doctors of alcohol-related problems is often identified as an obstacle to better treatment for problem drinkers. The Department organised a seminar on Alcohol-Related Problems in Higher

---

*1 Unit = ½ pint of ordinary beer or a standard measure of wine/spirits.

Professional and Post-graduate Medical Education. Medical Schools in England were surveyed to establish their current practice on teaching medical students about alcohol. A Conference on Alcohol Detoxification Services marked the publication of a review on this topic and brought together people in the field to discuss the way in which services should develop in the future. Most problem drinkers are in work and the special role of the workplace in prevention and detection of alcohol problems was emphasised by the Secretary of State in his speech to a Conference organised by ACCEPT (Addictions Community Centres for Education, Prevention Treatment and Research).

Prevention

All of these indications of the magnitude of the alcohol misuse problem highlight again the importance of preventing harm by promoting sensible drinking habits. At national level, the Government clearly has a role in this. The Secretary of State hosted a Departmental conference on Prevention of Alcohol Misuse attended by representatives of industry, advertising, media, treatment providers and organisations involved with young people.

At local level there is scope for a range of preventive activities. A useful practical guide appeared in the form of a book 'Preventing Alcohol Problems. A Guide to Local Action'[9] supported by Departmental funding.

Services

The Department produced guidelines for use by the Hospital Advisory Service (HAS) in the assessment of services for problem drinkers.

An experimental project for the detoxification of problem drinkers in their own homes is currently being evaluated in Exeter, supported by Departmental funding.

References

[1] Maynard A, Hardman G, Whelan A. Data note 9: measuring the social cost of addictive substances. *Brit J Addict* 1987, **82**: 701–6.
[2] Special Committee of the Royal College of Psychiatrists. Alcohol: our favourite drug: New report on alcohol and alcohol-related problems. London: Tavistock, 1986.
[3] Royal College of General Practitioners. Alcohol: a balanced view. Exeter: Royal College of General Practitioners, 1986. (Report from general practice; 24).
[4] Royal College of Physicians of London. A great and growing evil: the medical consequences of alcohol abuse. London: Tavistock, 1987.
[5] Parliamentary Group of the Standing Committee on Communications. *Psychological aspects of alcohol: a report prepared by the Parliamentary Group of the Standing Committee on Communications.* Leicester: British Psychological Society, 1986.
[6] British Medical Association Board of Science and Education. Young people and alcohol: British Medical Association, 1986.
[7] Marsh A, Dobbs Joy, White Amanda. Adolescent drinking: a survey carried out on behalf of the DHSS and the SHHD. London: HMSO, 1986.
[8] Orford J, Wawman T. Alcohol detoxification services: a review. DHSS (Stanmore), 1986.
[9] Tether P, Robinson D. Preventing alcohol problems: a guide to local action. London: Tavistock, 1986.

(g) Child abuse

The Department has completed a consultation exercise under the title 'Child Abuse — Working Together'. This has shown considerable support for the proposed procedures on inter-agency working. It is intended to publish this guidance, together with guidance in the handling of Child Abuse Inquiries, in 1987.

The Social Services Inspectorate report on the Supervision of Social Workers in the Assessment and Monitoring of Cases of Child Abuse[1] was issued in April 1986, and the Inspectorate are undertaking follow-up work with those agencies involved.

Recent statistics published by the National Society for the Prevention of Cruelty to Children (NSPCC)[2], who hold the Child Abuse Registers covering about 10% of the population, showed an overall increase of 42% in the number of children whose names were placed on these registers in one year. An increase of 126% in reported cases of child sexual abuse was noted.

Child sexual abuse
The statistics quoted in the previous section reflect at least in part an increased awareness of the problem of child sexual abuse, both by professionals and the public. One of the most pressing needs for professionals is for more and improved training on this subject at every level. To this end the Department has put in hand the first part of a strategy for training in the management of child sexual abuse. The training initiative was announced by the Secretary of State on 30 October 1986[3] — £100,000 is to be made available for each of 3 years to fund 2 training projects.

Firstly, to promote in-depth training, an additional training facility is to be funded at the Department of Psychological Medicine at the Hospital for Sick Children at Great Ormond Street. This proposal includes in-depth training and workshops. It is expected that trainees will be social workers, health visitors and medical practitioners seconded from different parts of the country. The hospital will train 6 people each year for 3 years, and the trainees are expected to be people who can develop their own skills to such an extent that they will be able to pass on what they learn within their own authority. A senior training lecturer is to be appointed.

Secondly, a Training Advisory Resource is to be based at the National Children's Bureau under the aegis of the Training Advisory Group on the Sexual Abuse of Children (TAGOSAC) formerly the CIBA group. The project is to stimulate multidisciplinary training for all types of practitioner by developing training materials and setting up an information resource. A project/development officer and a part-time Consultant will support the work of TAGOSAC.

It is hoped that these preliminary training initiatives will supplement both the specific training required for various professional groups, and facilitate the prevention and management of child sexual abuse. The Department's training strategy will be expanded in 1987, and will address child abuse generally.

A Department press release also announced DHSS support for 2 telephone counselling services.

43

(a) **Childline** — a national facility set up by the BBC Childwatch programme as a charity. The Department made a launching grant of £50,000.

(b) **Touchline** — an innovative local facility in Yorkshire for children and families, organised by the National Children's Home in consultation with Leeds Social Services. The Department has made a grant of £53,000 over 3 years, and the project will be evaluated.

It is hoped these ventures will offer help for older children suffering abuse, supported by back-up services.

References

[1] Pugh-Thomas R, Hey C, Ruber M, Woods G. *Inspection of the supervision of social workers in the assessment and monitoring of cases of child abuse when children, subject to a court order, have been returned home.* London (Alexander Fleming House, Elephant and Castle, SE1): Social Services Inspectorate, Headquarters. March 1986.

[2] National Society for the Prevention of Cruelty to Children. *Dramatic new child abuse figures.* Press release 9 December 1986.

[3] Department of Health and Social Security. *Government to provide £400,000 to combat child sexual abuse.* Press release 86/334, 30 October 1986.

3. ENVIRONMENTAL HEALTH

(a) Committee on the Medical Aspects of Radiation in the Environment (COMARE)

This Committee, which was established following a recommendation in the Black Advisory Group Report 'to advise Government on the medical aspects of radiation in the environment' met 5 times in 1986. It published its first report[1] on 'The implications of the new data on the releases from Sellafield in the 1950s for the conclusions of the report on the Investigation of the Possible Increased Incidence of Cancer in West Cumbria', in July 1986, and also gave advice to Government on the health effects of radon in houses in December 1986.

COMARE's First report

The Advisory Group chaired by Sir Douglas Black had asked the National Radiological Protection Board (NRPB) to calculate the doses that were likely to have been received by the young people resident in Seascale village since the 1950s. In order to enable NRPB to do this the Group had asked BNFL to make available to NRPB all relevant monitoring and discharge data since the Sellafield site had begun its operations in 1952. NRPB based their dose estimates[2] on these data and the Black Advisory Group in their report[3], published in July 1984, referring to risk estimates based on these data, concluded (para 6.12) that 'these calculations do not support the view that the radiation released from Sellafield was responsible for the observed incidence of leukaemia in Seascale and its neighbourhood. However, it is important to stress the unavoidable uncertainties on dose in this situation and the model we have used does not exclude other possibilities'.

Included in the data provided by BNFL were details of an incident occurring between 1954 and 1955 when an estimated 440 g of uranium oxide spent fuel cartridges had inadvertently been released to the atmosphere. Following publication of the report further information became available (initially from a worker employed at the site in the 1950s) which caused BNFL to revise their estimate of the magnitude of this release upwards by a factor of more than 40 to about 20 kg.

Such a large revision upwards of releases from the site naturally raised the question of the completeness of the data provided to the Black Advisory Group and the impact of these changed calculations on the conclusions of the Group.

BNFL therefore instituted a major review of information relating to Sellafield discharges and environmental monitoring in early years and passed all additional information to NRPB who recalculated the dose estimates[4]. The Government asked COMARE to consider the implications of these new data for the conclusions drawn in the Black Advisory Group Report.

In its first Report[1] the Committee concluded that the increased doses were still well below those that would readily explain the observed cases of leukaemia in Seascale, using conventional risk estimates. Thus the substance and essential conclusions of the Black Advisory Group Report remain unchanged.

(b) Radon in houses

In 1984 the Royal Commission on Environmental Pollution[5] recommended that the Government consider whether there was a need for action to reduce levels of the radioactive gas, radon, in certain houses. In 1986 the NRPB completed a survey of the levels of radon in houses in England and Wales; COMARE was asked for advice on the health implications of their results.

Radon gas is released to the environment from certain types of rocks by the decay of uranium. While the gas quickly disperses in the open air, quite high levels of radon can develop in confined spaces or where there is limited ventilation, such as inside houses, or mines. In such situations the radon gas is inhaled and irradiates the lungs. A number of studies of miners have demonstrated increased rates of lung cancer from exposure to radon gas.

COMARE advised that exposure to radon gas in some houses must be considered a public health problem. It agreed that the 'action level' of 20 mSv per year suggested by NRPB for existing houses was a reasonable starting point. The Committee indicated that the dosimetry and risk estimation procedure employed included many uncertainties which the Committee wished to address in more detail at a later date.

For new buildings the Committee recommended that exposures should be as consistent as possible with the internationally recommended dose limits regarding annual exposure to members of the public from all artificial sources of radiation.

The Committee also recommended that the feasibility of a study of the effects of radon exposure in dwellings in the UK on members of the public be considered. DHSS and the Department of the Environment (DOE) are considering the best way of taking this recommendation forward in consultation with COMARE and the NRPB.

Since levels of radon in the environment relate to the geology of the area, most of the houses in England with levels of radon gas above the 'action' level are likely to be found in Devon and Cornwall. NRPB, in consultation with the DOE is conducting a more detailed screening programme which is aimed at identifying these houses and advising on remedial measures that can be taken to reduce the levels. The DOE have also published an information leaflet[6] on the subject.

Other work in progress
In December 1985 a Yorkshire Television Programme suggested that there were excess rates of cancer in young children living near the Atomic Weapons Research establishments at Aldermaston, the Royal Ordnance Factory at Burghfield and the Nuclear Submarine bases at Faslane, Rosyth and Holy Loch and that this was linked to the presence of these establishments.

At about the same time the Information Services Division (now Information and Statistics Division) of the Scottish Health Services Common Services Agency made public the results of studies of leukaemia rates within Scotland including the areas round the reprocessing plant at Dounreay[7,8,9].

A number of other studies on cancer rates in children have been published recently, including an analysis by independent researchers of the OPCS statistics relating to areas around nuclear installations in England and Wales[10].

COMARE has been asked to advise on all of the above studies. Obviously, completing such an extensive programme of work will take some time, especially since at each site there is a need for site-specific discharge and environmental monitoring data to be collated and assessed. Furthermore, as is the case with Aldermaston and Burghfield, there is frequently a need for more detailed epidemilogical studies of the areas before any conclusions can be drawn.

Advice from COMARE on the cancer rates around Aldermaston and Burghfield is at present expected by the end of 1987.

(c) Chernobyl

During the night of 26 April 1986 a serious accident involving an explosion and fire took place in the Number 4 Nuclear Reactor at Chernobyl in Byelorussia in the USSR. The plume of radioactivity released during the following 10 days was dispersed over a large part of the western hemisphere during the next few weeks and resulted in variable quantities of radioactivity being deposited on the ground within Western Europe, including the UK. Over a year later the impact of this event is still being assessed.

The radioactive cloud reached the United Kingdom on 2 May and moved from the south east of England in a north-westerly direction. In areas where rain fell while the radioactive cloud was overhead, additional radioactivity was washed from the cloud onto the ground including grass and vegetables, and into the sea and inland waters.

While the cloud was overhead rain fell mainly in parts of Scotland, North West England (including Cumbria and the Isle of Man) and North Wales, so that these were generally the most affected areas within the UK.

The NRPB, supported by laboratories in the nuclear industry and relevant government departments, carried out extensive monitoring of levels of radionuclides in the air, in rainwater, on the ground and in food and milk, to form a basis for decisions on the need for intervention.

The radionuclides in the cloud that were detected in significant quantities in the UK were Iodine-131, Caesium-137 and Caesium-134. Other radionuclides (such as Strontium-89 and Strontium-90) were detected in countries closer to the accident.

The levels of radionuclides in cow's milk in the UK were carefully monitored over the following days since both iodine and caesium are secreted in milk. However, although these radionuclides were detected in cow's milk, the levels did not rise sufficiently for any action to be necessary.

The first action that was necessary was to advise against the drinking of 'undiluted' rainwater in the most affected areas between 3–8 May.

47

As an emergency measure on 1 May, DHSS advised Port Health Authorities to hold and test imports of fresh fruit, vegetables fish and dairy products exported from Poland and Russia after 26 April. This advice was later extended to include other Eastern bloc countries (Bulgaria, Czechoslovakia, Hungary, Rumania and Yugoslavia). On 13 May the European Council imposed by Regulation a temporary ban on the import of food into the Community from the same countries. The ban continued until 31 May when it was replaced by a further Regulation which introduced arrangements for the monitoring of imports into the European Community from third countries.

Under these arrangements food imported into the UK from the 7 countries previously mentioned plus Austria, East Germany, Sweden and Turkey continues to be monitored to check compliance with the European control ('action') levels of 370 becquerels per kilogram (Bq/kg) of caesium 134/137 for milk and baby foods and 600 Bq/kg for all other foods. These arrangements will continue until the expiry of the Regulation on 31 October 1987. The UK received information on similar monitoring being carried out in other member states.

In June the levels of radiocaesium in young lambs not yet ready for market in some areas of Cumbria, North Wales and Scotland were sufficiently high for the Government to decide to use its powers under the Food and Environment Protection Act 1985 to prohibit the movement and slaughter of sheep in the affected areas. This prevented the affected meat from entering the food chain. Initially 4.2 million sheep (out of a national flock of 24.6 million) were affected by the order. Although most of the affected areas have now been released, some 300,000 sheep (as of April 1987) still remain subject to control.

The Community experienced considerable difficulty in agreeing the 'action' level for their Regulation and internationally there has also been considerable debate on the question of acceptable levels of radionuclides in food following a nuclear accident.

The dose or exposure any person will receive from a given radionuclide in food will obviously depend on how much of the food is consumed. Therefore 'acceptable' levels in the same food can, in theory, vary from one country to another depending on variations in consumption rates, and also on the extent of the contamination of other foods. Similarly, acceptable levels of radioactivity in different foods can also in theory vary depending on whether the food is a major or minor component of the diet. However, for international purposes any system of controls has to be considerably simplified in order for it to be practical. Agreement on the criteria for this simplification has not been easy to achieve.

In this context it may be helpful to explain that the becquerel (Bq) measures the amount of radioactivity present in any item, while the sievert (Sv) measures the dose that is received from a given exposure to radiation. Because these units were unfamiliar to many people before Chernobyl, the fact that every year we receive on average two thousandths of a sievert (or two millisieverts) from natural background radiation (eg radon in the home and cosmic rays from outer space), and that in Devon and Cornwall exposures of over 10 times this level per year from radon in a small number of houses have been detected, may help to put things in context. A chest X-ray will give a dose of about a twentieth of natural background (0.1 mSv) to the lung. Average consumers of lamb would have received 0.15 mSv in the year if *all* the lamb they had consumed since Chernobyl had been contaminated at the maximum permitted level of 1000 Bq of caesium 134/137 per kilogram of lamb (which is very unlikely). NRPB have calculated that the average adult living in a high rainfall area is likely to have received 0.3 mSv over the last year from the consequences of Chernobyl[11]. It is therefore reassuring to find that the exposures in the UK as a result of Chernobyl have generally been small relative to background radiation.

There is, internationally, an appreciation of the fact that there were many areas where confusion arose because there was insufficient internationally agreed guidance on the management of such a severe nuclear accident. These problems are being addressed at present by a number of agencies including the World Health Organization (WHO), the International Atomic Energy Agency and the International Commission on Radiological Protection.

Immediately following Chernobyl a thorough review of the UK's contingency plans for dealing with nuclear accidents was instituted. The review concluded that existing plans continued to provide a valid basis for the response to any nuclear accident that occurred in the UK. However the Government decided planning was needed to provide more specifically for the responses to a nuclear accident outside the UK. This new plan is being developed as quickly as possible.

(d) Chlorination of drinking water

The normal disinfection of water by chlorination leads to the incidental formation of byproducts from traces of organic substances present in the source waters. Ingestion of large amounts of certain of the byproducts, such as some of the trihalomethanes (which include chloroform) is known to cause cancer in laboratory rodents. Furthermore, descriptive epidemiological studies conducted in the 1970s in the United States led to concern that the incidence of certain types of cancer in man might be increased by drinking-water containing the byproducts of chlorination. The later discovery that concentrated extracts of chlorinated water were mutagenic in bacterial assays added to the concern. In 1978, the Department's Joint Committee on Medical Aspects of Water Quality considered the trihalomethanes, and judged that

"the evidence concerning a carcinogenic risk, from current levels of trihalomethanes, is inconclusive but any risk which may exist is likely to be extremely small".

Since 1978 there has been much analytical, epidemiological and toxicological research on chlorination byproducts, some of which has taken place in the UK, along lines suggested by the Joint Committee, as part of the programme funded by the DOE in the area of water quality and health. The results were assessed in 1986 by the Committee on Medical Aspects of Contamination of Air, Soil and Water (which succeeded the Joint Committee in 1984). In August 1986, the Committee stated that

"We have found no sound reason to conclude that the consumption of the byproducts of chlorination, in drinking-water which has been treated and chlorinated according to current practices, increases the risk of cancer in humans".

The statement included recommendations for further research, designed in particular to elucidate the results of the mutagenicity assays, and this is in progress under funding from the DOE.

(e) Intolerance to food additives

In March 1987, the Food Advisory Committee of MAFF published its final report on colours in food[12]. The report includes an extensive evaluation of the toxicity of food colours by the DHSS Committee on Toxicity of Chemicals in Food, Consumer Products and the Environment (COT). One particular area addressed by the COT in the report is the question of intolerance to food additives including colours. While there is no scientific evidence that intolerance to food colours is an extensive problem, the COT was aware that this is nevertheless perceived as being a widespread phenomenon by many members of the public.

Adverse reactions have been reported in association with a wide range of foods and food ingredients, including food additives[13,14], but the prevalence of intolerance reactions has not been established. However, there is general agreement that intolerance reactions to foods and major food ingredients (such as cow's milk, eggs, wheat, fish, shellfish, citrus fruits, etc) are much more common, perhaps affecting up to 20% of the population at some time in their lives[13], compared with reactions to food additives which have been estimated to affect 0.03–0.15% of the population[15].

Although the proportion of people who show intolerance to certain additives is very small, the nature of the adverse reactions can be very unpleasant (for example urticaria, eczema, asthma and rhinitis). For those who have identified additives which provoke a reaction, the new labelling Regulations for foods, which came into full effect in July 1986 and require manufacturers to declare ingredients, including additives, on the label, will enable them to avoid foods containing those additives. The COT did not consider there was sufficient evidence that particular additives were more likely to cause adverse reactions than other additives, and thought there were therefore no grounds for taking any special action beyond that already undertaken on labelling of foods. An extensive research project commissioned by MAFF is now underway, which has as its initial aim the assessment of the likely prevalence of adverse reactions to food additives among the population at large. We will be reviewing our advice on this matter when the results of this study become available.

(f) Novel foods

One potentially important development in agricultural science and food technology is the possibility of producing novel foods for human consumption. A novel food can be defined as a food wholly or largely composed of material which has not hitherto been used for human consumption, or which has been produced using new processes not previously used in the production of food. Examples are foods made from single cell organisms such as bacteria or fungi; these organisms are typically grown in and harvested from large industrial fermentation vessels, and are then processed, coloured and flavoured to produce items which look and taste similar to traditional foods such as meat products. One such food derived from single cell organisms has been given Ministerial clearance and is available on the UK retail food market.

In the near future it is likely that the techniques of biotechnology, including the use of genetic manipulation, will be increasingly applied to novel foods. For example, there is a possibility of using genetically modified yeasts in the brewing and baking industries, or of applying genetic engineering to produce new varieties of traditional food crops which will have improved pest or frost resistance. Another possibility is the use of recombinant DNA techniques to produce veterinary medicines or other products used in animal husbandry; for example bovine growth hormone derived from genetically modified bacteria which could be used in the rearing of beef cattle.

All these developments offer the possibility of economic and other advantages to the consumer and industry. But, like other examples of technological innovation, they also raise questions about how the safety of the new products can be assured. A novel food may contain novel chemical substances which might present a toxicological hazard to the consumer. Novel foods may also differ in important nutritional respects from the traditional foods which they may replace, and could possibly have an unfavourable impact on the nutritional status of consumers. Finally there is the possibility that novel foods might pose special microbiological problems for consumers.

In 1982 Ministers appointed the Advisory Committee on Irradiated and Novel Foods (ACINF) to advise Health and Agriculture Ministers on matters relating to food irradiation or to the manufacture of novel foods. In the UK there exists a voluntary scheme whereby any company which is proposing to develop or import a product which appears to fall within the definition of a novel food is requested to notify MAFF. If necessary the company will be advised to seek formal Ministerial clearance, in which case all the data on the product will be submitted to ACINF, who may also seek the advice of other expert committees before reaching a conclusion. ACINF will advice Ministers of its conclusions and, if appropriate, a formal Ministerial clearance for the new product will be issued.

The ACINF has issued guidelines[16] specifying the type of safety data which companies should produce in support of any application for Ministerial clearance, and indicating how the committee will evaluate those data. If necessary ACINF will refer nutritional questions to the COMA Panel on Novel Foods. They have terms of reference which include the consideration of the nutritional aspects of any novel food or food process submitted by manufacturers. COMA advised in 1972 that any substance promoted as a replacement or alternative to a natural food should be the nutritional equivalent in all but unimportant aspects of the food it would simulate. In 1980 this advice was extended to require that novel foods intended to simulate meat should contain the major nutrients provided by meat — namely protein quantity and quality, thiamin and vitamin B_{12} — and that iron should be added to bring the substitute to a specified level.

At present the development of novel foods has only recently begun to make an impact in the food industry. However, the fact that procedures already exist which allow the proper safety evaluation of these products means that these potentially beneficial technological developments can occur without raising fears about adverse consequences for human health.

References

1 Bobrow M. First report: the implications of the new data on the releases from Sellafield in the 1950s for the conclusions of the Report on the Investigations of the possible increased incidence of cancer in West Cumbria. London: HMSO, 1986.

2 Stather J W, Wrixon A D, Simmonds J R. The risks of leukaemia and other cancers in Seascale from radiation exposure. NRPB Report R-171 Chilton, sold by HMSO, 1984.

3 Black D. Investigation of the possible increased incidence of cancer in West Cumbria: report of the Independent Advisory Group. London: HMSO, 1984.

4 Stather J W, Dionian J, Brown J, Fell T P, Muirhead C R. The risks of leukaemia and other cancer in Seascale from radiation exposure: addendum to report R-171 Chilton: National Radiological Protection Board, sold by HMSO, 1986.

5 Royal Commission on Environmental Pollution. Tackling pollution: experience and prospects: tenth report. London: HMSO, 1984.

6 Department of the Environment. *Radon in houses*. London: Department of the Environment, 1987.

7 Heasman M *et al*. Childhood leukaemia in N Scotland. *Lancet* 1986; **i:** 266 and **i:** 385.

8 Heasman M *et al*. Leukaemia in young persons in Scotland. A study of its geographical distributions and relationship to nuclear installations. *Hlth Bull* 1987; **45:** 3 (May).

9 Information Services Division of Scottish Health Services Common Services Agency. In Evidence to Inquiry related to Planning Application for a European Demonstration Fast Reactor Fuel Reprocessing Plant at Dounreay. Caithness, 1986.

10 Cook-Mozaffari P J, Ashwood F L, Vincent T, Forman D, Alderson M. Cancer incidence and mortality in the vicinity of nuclear installations: England and Wales, 1959–80. London: HMSO, 1987. (Studies on medical and population subjects; no 51).

11 Morrey M, Brown J, Williams J A, Crick M J, Simmonds J R, Hill M D. A preliminary assessment of the radiological impact of the Chernobyl reactor accident on the population of the European Community. National Radiological Protection Board, 1987.

12 Food Advisory Committee, Ministry of Agriculture, Fisheries and Food. Final report on the review of Colouring Matter in Food Regulations 1973. London: HMSO, 1987.

13 Royal College of Physicians of London and the British Nutrition Foundation. Food intolerance and food aversion: a joint report of the Royal College of Physicians and the British Nutrition Foundation. London: Royal College of Physicians, 1984.

14 National Institute of Allergy and Infectious Diseases. American Academy of Allergy and Immunology: Committee on Adverse Reactions to Foods. *Adverse reactions to foods*, Washington DC: Department of Health and Human Services, 1984.

15 Commission of the European Communities. *Report of the Scientific Committee for Food (12th series), 1981*. Brussels: Commission of the European Communities, 1982: Annex p. 5 (EUR 7823).

16 Department of Health and Social Security, Ministry of Agriculture, Fisheries and Food, Scottish Home and Health Department, Welsh Office, Department of Health and Social Services, Northern Ireland. Memorandum on the testing of novel foods, incorporating guidelines for testing. Advisory Committee on Irradiated and Novel Foods. London: MAFF, 1984.

4. COMMUNICABLE DISEASES

(a) Acquired immune deficiency syndrome (AIDS) and HIV infection

In 1986 there was a rapid escalation of public awareness of AIDS, and both in the UK and world wide the numbers of reported cases increased considerably. Moves were made towards international co-operation in tackling the problem of infection with the AIDS virus. This retro virus in early 1986 was still known by a variety of names, commonly HTLV III or LAV. In May 1986 the International Committee on Taxonomy of Viruses decided that the virus should henceforth be known as The Human Immune Deficiency Virus (HIV).

(i) Surveillance

In the UK AIDS and HIV infection is not a notifiable disease. The reason for this is that at present statutory notification would not facilitate prevention of spread nor increase the completeness of case ascertainment. Furthermore it is possible that in common with other sexually transmitted diseases anxieties about the maintenance of confidentiality might discourage patients with HIV from coming forward for advice if the condition were made statutorily notifiable.

The voluntary reporting system for AIDS cases set up by the Communicable Disease Surveillance Centre (CDSC) in 1982 continues to operate[1]. In England the clinician in charge of an AIDS patient reports the case in strict confidence to CDSC. Deaths ascribed to AIDS are also reported and provide a cross-check.

With regard to tests positive for anti-bodies to HIV all Public Health Laboratory Service (PHLS) laboratories in England, Wales and Northern Ireland report their results to the CDSC. NHS and private laboratories are also encouraged to make reports to CDSC. A small sample of laboratories report both positive and negative test. The information thus obtained provides incomplete evidence of the extent of HIV infection in the population. The results are also biased. For example, it is very probable that a larger proportion of haemophiliacs have been tested than is the case for, say, intravenous drug misuers.

(ii) AIDS

In the UK in 1986 there were 339 cases of AIDS reported of which 298 were reported from England. This brought the cumulative total in the UK to 578 at 31 December 1986 of which 551 were reported from England (Table 4.1). As may be seen from Table 4.1 the bulk of cases have been concentrated in the Thames Regions, notably in NW Thames.

The number of AIDS cases reported by the USA continued to dominate the international situation in 1986 with a total of 13,008 cases being notified to the Centre for Disease Control, Atlanta. WHO received reports[2] of AIDS cases from an increasing number of member states. In interpreting these reports it is necessary to recognise that reporting systems in some countries are rudimentary and that in many countries the facilities for diagnosing AIDS are very poor. It is widely recognised that the AIDS epidemic has reached major

Table 4.1: *England — Reports of AIDS to 31 December 1986 by Region of reporter*

Region	New cases (1986)	Cumulative total to 31 December 1986	Percentage of total reports
Northern	10	18	3
Yorkshire	7	7	1
Trent	8	10	2
East Anglia	3	5	1
N W Thames	149	274	50
N E Thames	44	103	19
S E Thames	36	52	9
S W Thames	5	14	3
Wessex	3	13	2
Oxford	4	6	1
South Western	2	9	2
West Midlands	8	12	2
Mersey	5	7	1
North Western	14	21	4
Total	298	551	100

Table 4.2: *AIDS cases up to 31 December 1986 in various European countries (as reported to WHO by 1 June 1987), comparable USA figures are given at the foot of the table*

Country	Population (million)	Cases reported for 1986	Cumulative cases to 31 December 1986	Cumulative cases per million population to 31 December 1986
Belgium	9.9	55	216	21.9
Denmark	5.1	59	131	25.5
France	54.6	648	1,221	22.4
Italy	56.9	343	539	9.5
Netherlands	14.5	112	218	15.0
Spain	39.0	134	264	6.8
W Germany	61.1	445	914	15.0
UK	56.0	311	577	10.3
USA	230	13,008	29,003	126.0

proportions in parts of central, east, and southern Africa, yet at the end of December 1986 the cumulative totals of cases reported to WHO form all of Africa was only 3,334.

The cumulative total reported from Europe up to 31 December 1986 was 4,577 of which 2,350 cases were reported in 1986. Table 4.2 shows the cumulative incidence rates in selected European countries. The cumulative incidence rate of AIDS in the USA is shown for comparison.

In England in common with many European countries and the United States by far the largest group of cases of AIDS is in homosexual and bisexual men (Table 4.3) and the sex ratio is 33:1. This contrasts with the experience in

Africa where the ratio of males to females affected is approximately 1:1[3], and with Scotland and some other European countries where the proportion of AIDS cases who are intravenous drug abusers is much higher[4]. The cumulative incidence of AIDS in England increases with age to the age-group 35–44 years after which it declines (Table 4.4).

(iii) HIV infection

By the end of 1986 2,150 individuals with positive tests for HIV anti-bodies had been reported in England. As for AIDS cases the largest group were homosexual or bisexual males (Table 4.5), but substantial numbers of positive tests in haemophiliacs, and intravenous drug abusers were also reported. In

Table 4.3: *Cumulative totals of reports of AIDS cases in England by transmission characteristic to 31 December 1986*

Transmission characteristics	Number of cases Male	Female	Total	Percentage
Homosexual/bisexual	488	0	488	88.6
Intravenous drug abuser (IVDA)	5	1	6	1.1
Homosexual & IVDA	7	0	7	1.3
Haemophiliac	21	0	21	3.8
Recipient of blood				
— abroad	3	3	6	1.1
— UK	2	1	3	0.5
Heterosexual:				
presumed infected abroad	7	4	11	2.0
presumed infected in UK	0	3	3	0.5
Child of HIV positive mother	1	2	3	0.5
Other	1	2	3	0.5
Total	535	16	551	99.9*

* Total does not add up to 100 because of rounding.

Table 4.4: *Cumulative total of AIDS cases in England by age to 31 December 1986 (both sexes)*

Age Group	Estimated population at mid 1986 (millions)	Number of cases	No of cases per million estimated population
0 – 14	8.9	5	0.6
15 – 24	7.7	24	3.1
25 – 34	6.8	61	23.7
35 – 44	6.5	09	32.2
45 – 54	5.1	92	18.0
55 – 64	5.1	23	14.5
65 – +	7.3	6	1.2
Age unknown	—	31	—
Totals	47.4	551	11.6

Table 4.5: *HIV positive cases reported in England in 1986 by transmission characteristics*

Transmission characteristics	Male	Female	Unknown	Total	(%)
Homo/bisexual	1,265	0	0	1,265	(59)
IVDA	117	58	4	179	(8.5)
Homo/IVDA	14	0	0	14	(0.5)
Haemophilia	404	1	0	405	(19)
Recipient of blood	16	10	0	26	(1)
Heterosexual contact					
a) of above groups	5	27	0	32	(1.5)
b) of other groups	30	14	1	45	(2)
c) no information	0	0	0	0	(0)
Child of HIV+ mother	5	3	1	9	(0.5)
Several risks	3	0	0	3	(0)
No information	159	12	9	180	(8)
Total	2,010	125	15	2,150	100

84% of the persons with positive tests there was insufficient information on which to assign them to a risk group. However as almost all of these were men it is likely that most were homosexuals or bisexuals.

The situation in England contrasts with that of Scotland, which has been the source of some 20% of the HIV positive cases reported in the UK. In Scotland there is a high proportion of intravenous drug abusers among the cases reported as HIV positive and about a quarter are women[4]. This is also seen in some other European countries, notably Italy and Spain[5]. It increases the potential for heterosexual transmission of HIV. Infected women can pass the virus to their unborn children.

Table 4.6: *Cumulative totals of HIV positive cases reported in England by region of reporter to 31 December 1986*

Region	Number of cases	(% of total)
Northern	195	(9)
Yorkshire	81	(4)
Trent	97	(4.5)
East Anglia	47	(2)
N W Thames	685	(32)
N E Thames	311	(14.5)
S E Thames	305	(14)
S W Thames	55	(3)
Wessex	102	(5)
Oxford	66	(3)
South Western	57	(3)
West Midlands	67	(3)
Mersey	27	(1)
North Western	55	(2)
Total	2,150	(100)

Table 4.6 shows the regional distribution of HIV positive cases reported in England to 31 December 1986. As for AIDS cases these are concentrated in the Thames regions but the relative contribution of other regions is greater than it is for AIDS cases.

Although undoubtedly some individuals are tested in regions other than those in which they live, which distorts the picture, there is no question but that the infection is spreading.

(iv) Measures taken to prevent the spread of HIV infection

In the absence of any effective vaccine or cure prevention of the spread of the underlying virus infection is the only strategy for dealing with AIDS.

Public education campaign
In March 1986 a campaign was launched with the aim of informing the public about AIDS, the ways by which the infection is and is not transmitted and how to protect themselves and others.

The initial phase involved advertisements in the national press, the publication of a leaflet from the HEC[6] and the establishment of a telephone service, which was run by the College of Health and funded by the DHSS. In addition, the Terrance Higgins Trust and the Standing Conference on Drug Abuse (SCODA) produced posters and leaflets and there were advertisements in the gas press. An interim evaluation of the Department's campaign in July 1986 revealed it had widespread support and further advertisements were placed in the national press. In November 1986 the campaign was greatly widened and intensified, newspaper advertising was increased and a campaign aimed at young people was started through magazines, cinema and radio advertisements.

The DHSS leaflet *'Protect your Health Abroad'* was revised to include a section on AIDS[7].

In April 1987 the HEC was reconstituted as a Special Health Authority and was given major executive responsibility for public education about AIDS (see p. 31).

Voluntary bodies
Throughout 1986 the involvement of voluntary organisations in AIDS related matters increased. The bodies have an important role in complementing statutory provision. In particular they can provide information to those in high risk groups and counselling and support services for people who are HIV positive or have AIDS. The largest voluntary organisation solely concerned with AIDS is the Terrence Higgins Trust. In addition there is a growing number of specialist bodies such as the Haemophilia Society and SCODA which provide support for particular categories of high risk individuals.

Needle exchange programmes
The spread of HIV infection among intravenous drug abusers is attributable to the practice of sharing injecting equipment.

In December 1986 it was announced that schemes would be set up in 1987 whereby drug abusers could exchange used needles and syringes for clean ones in an attempt to reduce equipment sharing.

Professional guidelines
In January and June 1986 letters were sent to all doctors in England dealing with problems relating to AIDS in children at school.

In April 1986 guidance was issued for surgeons, anaesthetists and dentists in relation to HIV infected patients and in July 1986 guidance for doctors about artificial insemination was published.

In addition DHSS guidelines were issued in 1986 concerning HIV antibody testing of blood donations outside the National Blood Transfusion Service (NBTS), planning in the health services and AIDS in relation to local authority staff.

In June The Advisory Committee on Dangerous Pathogens (ACDP) presented a revision of the guidelines it first produced in December 1984[7-17].

AIDS and blood transfusion
The screening of all blood donations collected by the NBTS for HIV antibody was first introduced in October 1985. Between January and December 1986 2,625,385 donations were tested, and 54 were confirmed positive (0.002%). From February 1986 a separate record was kept of donations given by newly recruited volunteers. During the year some 391,698 donations were received and 18 of these were confirmed as HIV antibody positive (0.004%).

All donors, 44 men and 10 women, who were confirmed positive have been asked to attend Regional Transfusion Centres where they have been interviewed by medical staff who have been specially trained to counsel patients with HIV infection. With the exception of 2 male donors all responded to recall. All but 4 of those interviewed admitted to being in high-risk groups.

A revised leaflet for blood donors was issued in September 1986[18]. Its purpose was to describe more explicitly the risk groups and in particular to emphasise the risk posed by the heterosexual nature of infection in Africa, so as to ensure that people who have been exposed to such risks would exclude themselves from donating blood. The rate of positive donors found in the UK is comparable to that found in volunteer donors in Scandinavian countries, and substantially lower than that in many other European countries or in the United States.

Blood products
During 1986 heat-treated coagulation factors both from commercial sources and supplied by the Blood Products Laboratory (BPL), Elstree, were made from plasma which had been screened for HIV antibody.

ACDP guidelines
Revised guidelines were published by ACDP providing health care staff with a review of AIDS in general and giving specific recommendations for precautions to be taken by health care workers when handling specimens believed to be or known to be infected with HIV[13]. More than 70,000 copies of

these guidelines have now been issued and have been well received. The steadily accruing epidemiological evidence on routes of transmission of AIDS infection allowed emphasis to be placed on the need to avoid needlestick injury. There was a lack of evidence that the infection was spread by airborne virus particles. Up to the end of 1986 there are only 4 health care workers who have seroconverted following accidents (all involving hypodermic needles), compared with many hundreds of recorded incidents of exposure to HIV infected blood, body fluids and needlestick injury in which there is evidence that the person who sustained the injury did not become infected.

The CDSC has records of over 150 incidents involving needlestick or contamination of mucous membranes in British health care workers. In only one case did the person concerned (a nurse) become infected.

HN(86)25 HIV antibody in diagnostic reagents[17]
Following concern expressed to the DHSS that quality control and calibration materials and other diagnostic reagents used in pathology laboratories might be contaminated with HIV the DHSS issued advice to the NHS on the purchase of such materials.

After consultation with the NHS and the manufacturers of the materials an implementation date of 1 January 1987 was set after which laboratories were recommended to purchase, where possible, only materials which had been tested at source for HIV antibody as individual donations, or had been treated to inactivate any possible HIV virus. Specific, short-term, exceptions were allowed for certain rare materials. At the same time advice was given to laboratories on the use of materials derived from volunteers and patients for quality control purposes. The UK was the first country to issue such detailed advice on HIV in diagnostic reagents. It should be emphasised that no case of infection in laboratory staff resulting from the use of these essential products has been reported, and it cannot be said often enough that within laboratories good standards of practice are the most effective method of reducing risk of infection from either HIV or any other contaminant of body fluids.

(v) New human retroviruses

The emergence of two apparently new human retroviruses was reported in 1986. LAV 2 and HTLV IV were described by French and American investigators respectively. LAV 2 was identified in patients with AIDS or an AIDS-like illness who were of West African origin. In contrast HTLV IV has so far been found only in health subjects in Senegal. The degree of similarity between these two viruses is only now becoming clear but importantly they are both reported to be more closely related to a known monkey retrovirus (STLV III) than to HIV (HTLV III/LAV). No person infected with either of these retroviruses has so far been identified within the UK. However, the situation with regard to blood donor screening is being kept under review.

(vi) Research

During 1986 there were major developments in the AIDS research programme by the MRC and the Departments of Health.

The main medical programme of Government — funded research into AIDS — was co-ordinated by the MRC through their Working Party on AIDS. The

Council works closely with the Health Departments who were represented on the Working Party. In December 1985, the Health Departments agreed to contribute jointly up to £295,000 per annum towards the cost of the UK Centre for the co-ordination of epidemiological research on AIDS, which was to be set up by the MRC. DHSS agreed to contribute up to £250,000 annually and the first payment was made in December 1986.

In January 1986 the MRC had awarded 6 grants and by December this number had increased to 21. Two of these are jointly funded with DHSS and a further 7 are supported from the Health Departments' contribution towards epidemiological studies. During the year the Council were able to fund all research proposals on AIDS submitted to them which met the necessary scientific criteria and standards. In December 1986 the DES allocated an additional £1m per year to the Council to enable it to continue the expansion of its AIDS research programme. At the end of 1986, the MRC put forward a suggestion for a direct programme of research to develop a vaccine to prevent infection and anti-viral drugs to treat those infected with the AIDS virus. Early in 1987 the Government allocated an additional £14.5m for this directed programme.

DHSS has also been able to fund all suitable research projects on AIDS in 1986 and by the end of the financial year had funded research to a total value of £260,000 in addition to the contribution made to the MRC programme. The projects funded by the Department include studies of the cost of services for patients with AIDS, behavioural studies of homosexual males, and effective ways of providing counselling for HIV antibody positive people. It was also agreed to fund an evaluation of the Needle Exchange Schemes for drug misusers. The DHSS Procurement Directorate has funded research into the screening of blood and donors for the AIDS virus and the Department's Health Building Directorate has undertaken background research on the accommodation required by patients with AIDS.

In December the Chief Scientist held the first meeting of the group that he has set up to review the Government-funded research programme. This was attended by Government Departments, research councils and Government agencies funding research in this area.

By the end of the year, many research groups and university departments had put forward suggestions for health services research and these ideas were to be considered for funding by DHSS in 1987.

(vii) Zidovudine ('*Retrovir*')

This drug, otherwise known as azidothymidine (AZT) was first developed in 1964 by American researchers as an anti-cancer drug, but showed no promise. In 1984, the United States subsidiary of Burroughs Wellcome developed it as an anti-viral agent for the treatment of AIDS. It inhibits the enzyme, reverse transcriptase, necessary for replication of retroviruses such as HIV, arrests the infection and improves the health of people with AIDS but it does not provide a cure.

In trials in the United States, it has been shown to prolong life, arrest weight loss and increase the well-being of people with AIDS. The treatment reduces the frequency of opportunistic infections and may also lead to improvements in the laboratory tests for immunodeficiency. Zidovudine also produces adverse effects in a high proportion of patients, including severe anaemia which may require blood transfusion. To sustain benefit treatment must be continued indefinitely.

In 1986 zidovudine was used in a few patients in England in clinical trial. There is a shortage of zidovudine but by the end of 1986 the Wellcome Foundation Ltd were increasing supplies and considering its application, licensing and distribution.

References

[1] Anonymous. Availability of informational material on AIDS [Editorial]. *NNWR* 1987; **35:** 819–20.

[2] World Health Organization. Acquired Immunodeficiency Syndrome (AIDS): global data. *Weekly Epidemiological Record* 1987; **no 11:** 74.

[3] Quiin T C, Mann J M, Curran J W, Piot P. AIDS in Africa: an epidemiologic paradigm. *Science* 1986; **234:** 955–63.

[4] Scottish Committee on HIV Infection and Intravenous Drug Misuse. *HIV infection in Scotland: report of the Scottish Committee on HIV Infection and Intravenous Drug Misuse.* Edinburgh: Scottish Home and Health Department, 1986.

[5] World Health Organization. Acquired Immunodeficiency Syndrome (AIDS): Situation in the WHO European Region as of 30 September 1986. *Weekly Epidemiological Record* 1987; **no 5:** 23–5.

[6] Health Education Council. *AIDS: what everybody needs to know.* London: Health Education Council, 1986.

[7] Department of Health and Social Security. *Protect your health abroad: vital information for people travelling overseas — especially hotter climates.* London: Department of Health and Social Security, 1986; DHSS leaflet SA35/1987.

[8] Department of Health and Social Security. *Children at school and problems related to AIDS.* London: Department of Health and Social Security, 1986; DHSS circular CMO(86)1; CNO(86)1.

[9] Department of Health and Social Security. *HTLV III antibody testing of blood donations outside the National Blood Transfusion Service (NBTS).* London: Department of Health and Social Security, 1986; DHSS circular DA(86)1.

[10] Department of Health and Social Security. *Health services development: resources assumptions and planning guidelines.* London: Department of Health and Social Security, 1986; DHSS circular HC(86)2; LAC(86)4.

[11] Department of Health and Social Security. *Guidance for surgeons, anaesthetists, dentists and their teams in dealing with patients infected with HTLV III.* London: Department of Health and Social Security, 1986; Enclosure to DHSS circular CMO(86)7. (Acquired Immune Deficiency Syndrome (AIDS): booklet 3).

[12] Department of Education and Science. *Children at school and problems relating to AIDS.* London: Department of Education and Science, 1986; DES administrative memorandum 2/86. (Enclosure to DHSS circular CMO(86)10).

[13] Advisory Committee on Dangerous Pathogens. *LAV/HTLV III: the causative agent of AIDS and related conditions: revised guidelines.* London: Department of Health and Social Security; Health and Safety Executive, 1986; Enclosure to DHSS circular HN(86)20; LASSL(86)7.

[14] Department of Health and Social Security. *Acquired Immune Deficiency Syndrome (AIDS) and artificial insemination: guidance for doctors and AI clinics.* London: Department of Health and Social Security, 1986; Enclosure to DHSS circular CMO(86)12. (AIDS booklet 4).

[15] Department of Health and Social Security. *Information and guidance on AIDS (Acquired Immune Deficiency Syndrome) for local authority staff.* London: Department of Health and Social Security, 1986; DHSS circular LASSL(86)8.

[16] Department of Health and Social Security. *AIDS: the acquired immune deficiency syndrome and HIV: the AIDS virus.* London: Department of Health and Social Security, 1986; DHSS circular CMO(86)18; CNO(86)18.

[17] Department of Health and Social Security. *HIV (LAV/HTLV III — "AIDS virus") antibody in diagnostic reagents and quality control and calibration materials.* London: Department of Health and Social Security, 1986; DHSS circular HN(86)25.

[18] National Blood Transfusion Service. *AIDS: what you must know before you give blood.* London: National Blood Transfusion Service, 1986. (NBTS 1181).

(b) Measles

Although there was a slight reduction (12.3%) in the total number of cases of measles notified in 1986 as compared with 1985, 82,072 cases of this preventable disease were notified, and many thousands more which were not notified occurred. The immunisation rate improved from 63% in 1985 to 68% in 1986. Nevertheless both this average figure and the substantial variation between Districts remains unsatisfactory.

(c) Rubella

In 1986 laboratory reports confirmed 196 cases of rubella infection in pregnancy. Many of the pregnancies were terminated[1]. Figure 4.1 shows the number of such cases for the period 1975–86.

In 1983 and 1984 pregnancy was terminated in 537 women who had been associated with rubella — 295 women had or were suspected of having rubella, 77 had been in contact with rubella and 165 had been inadvertently vaccinated against rubella shortly before or during their pregnancy. More than half these terminations (51%) were in parous women for whom opportunities had existed to identify their susceptibility to rubella.

These findings and other evidence prompted the Joint Committee on Vaccination and Immunisation to recommend that the present policy about rubella vaccination should be augmented by the introduction of a combined vaccine against measles, mumps and rubella (MMR) to be given to children of both sexes at the age of 15 months.

In order to encourage immunisation the National Rubella Council produced audio-visual material entitled 'Why worry?' for presentation to women's groups and a video aimed at teenage girls.

(d) Whooping cough

Notifications of whooping cough in 1986 (an epidemic year) were 36,500. Four deaths occurred. Although notifications were just over half those recorded in the equivalent epidemic years of 1978 and 1982, and the autumn peak observed in previous epidemic years, did not occur[2], it is to be hoped that no further epidemics of pertussis will occur within the UK. This will depend on further inprovements in the rate of immunisation. Nevertheless, strenuous efforts are needed to increase vaccination and break the 4-year epidemic cycle. The European Region of the WHO has suggested a target for uptake of pertussis vaccine of 90% by 1990.

(e) Poliomyelitis

Five patients with paralytic poliomyelitis were reported in 1986. Three of these appeared to be vaccine-associated:

(i) A 23-year-old married unimmunised man developed bulbar poliomyelitis. His son had been given oral poliovaccine 47 days before the onset of his father's illness;

Figure 4.1: *Laboratory confirmed rubella infections in pregnancy reported to the Communicable Disease Surveillance Centre, 1975-86*, England and Wales*

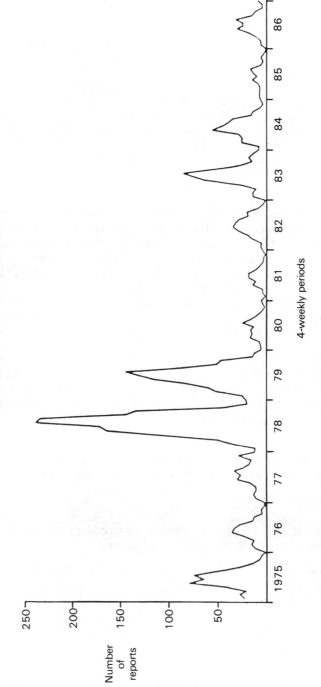

*Reprinted with permission from the British Medical Journal

(ii)   A 15-year-old schoolboy developed an influenza-like illness 12 days and unilateral footdrop 22 days after receiving a booster dose of oral poliovaccine. This patient had not travelled abroad; and

(iii)   Fifteen days after receiving her first dose of oral poliovaccine neurological signs which were not initially typical of poliomyelitis were noted in a 3-month old girl. Later lower motor neurone signs developed in all four limbs. The patient developed difficulty in breathing and died in spite of being ventilated. There was no laboratory evidence of poliomyelitis infection.

The other two cases do not appear to have been vaccine-associated. An unvaccinated 3-year-old boy acquired paralytic poliomyelitis after a visit to Pakistan. The second case was an unimmunised 62-year-old woman who became ill and later developed paresis of her upper and lower limbs and bulbar paralysis. This patient had not been abroad and had no history of close contact with young children.

(f) Diphtheria

Two cases of diphtheria, both imported from abroad were reported in 1986. The first was in an unimmunised 14-month-old child who was admitted to hospital with a two-day history of cough and stridor. On examination under anaesthetic the child was found to have a white membrane in the pharynx extending into the trachea. Culture of a throat swab yielded a toxigenic strain of *Corynebacterium diphtheriae*. The child had arrived in the UK from Bangladesh with her parents and 5 siblings. Four family members were found to be carriers of the toxigenic strain — 3 siblings (all of whom had injected fauces) and the father (who was asymptomatic).

Diphtheria was also diagnosed in a 31-year-old man from the West Midlands. He developed a sore throat and a throat swab, taken 4 days later, yielded a culture of a toxigenic *Corynebacterium diphtheriae*. His immunisation history could not be confirmed. Three days before the onset of his illness the patient, a long distance lorry driver, had given a lift to a hitch-hiker recently returned from Greece.

The hitch-hiker was subsequently traced but swabs taken were negative for *Corynebacterium diphtheriae*. The source of this infection was not found.

(g) Influenza

The winter of 1985–86 was the eighth successive season where there had been no increase of the epidemic indices for influenza.

Advice was issued to doctors in August 1986 concerning the composition of trivalent vaccine to be used for the next winter[3]. However, the appearance of strains of influenza A virus H1N1, which were significantly different from those in the current vaccine, prompted further advice on the use of a monovalent vaccine, which contained these new strains[4].

(h) Rabies

In mid-June 1986, a 46-year-old British woman residing in Lusaka, Zambia, was bitten on the arm and forearm when she attempted to break-up a fight between her guard dog and a stray dog which broke into the compound of her home. The woman did not seek medical advice following the injuries because she thought she had been bitten by her own dog which had been immunised against rabies. She travelled to the UK to visit her family 2 weeks later and remained in good health until 9 August when she complained of extensive fatigue. Two days later she developed fever, flu-like symptoms and bradycardia, all of which resolved in 24 hours. However, over the next 3 days her condition deteriorated with recurrent fever and hallucinations.

By 15 August a history of progressive hydrophobia led to a clinical diagnosis of rabies and the patient remained under sedation on a ventilator. She died 14 days later on 29 August. Clinical diagnosis was confirmed by isolation of viruses from saliva and post-mortem brain tissue.

About 50 contacts were traced and post-exposure vaccination given where necessary. Although a small theoretical risk of rabies transmission via body fluids exists, person to person transmission of rabies does not normally occur. Strict barrier nursing, with gowns, gloves and goggles was followed and staff caring for the patient received a pre-exposure vaccination course.

In the UK the control of rabies is based on preventing the entry of animals with rabies. This policy has been remarkably successful since 1902 when the last indigenous case of rabies were reported in Wales. The case reported above is the eighteenth imported case of human rabies reported in the UK since the beginning of the century. Most cases have followed dog bites in the Indian sub-continent, the only exceptions being one case in Indonesia and the case described above.

(i) Meningococcal meningitis

There were 858 notifications of meningococcal meningitis in 1986. Figure 4.2 shows the 5-week rolling average number of cases notified to OPCS between 1984 and 8 May 1987.

While the incidence of all meningococcal infection increased, the increase of non-typable Group B organisms was disproportionate (from 24% in 1985 to 41% in 1986). But the most notable change in prevalence has been the increase in Group C organisms rising from 16.7% in 1977 to 40.3% in 1986 (Table 4.7).

Particularly high rates of meningococcal infection continued to be reported for some communities. Since 1981, Gloucester Health District has experienced an outbreak due to Group B15 sulphonamide-resistant organisms with 89 cases between 1 October 1981 and 31 December 1986 (an incidence of 5.7/100,000 per annum compared with national average notification rate of 1/100,000 per annum). A DHSS-sponsored project began in November 1986 to investigate the prevalence of carriers of and immunity to Group B Type 15 sulphonamide-resistant meningococci in the parish of Stonehouse in Gloucestershire. Samples were obtained from 98% of the 77% of Stonehouse residents who took part for bacteriological, salivary and blood analysis. The first two reports of this study will be published in the *Journal of Epidemiology and Infection* in December 1987. There was low prevalence of Group B15 Pi16 Sulphonamide-resistant strains in the community of Stonehouse at a time when it was

Figure 4.2: *Meningococcal meningitis: 1984-1987 (May) England and Wales Notifications: 5-week rolling averages*

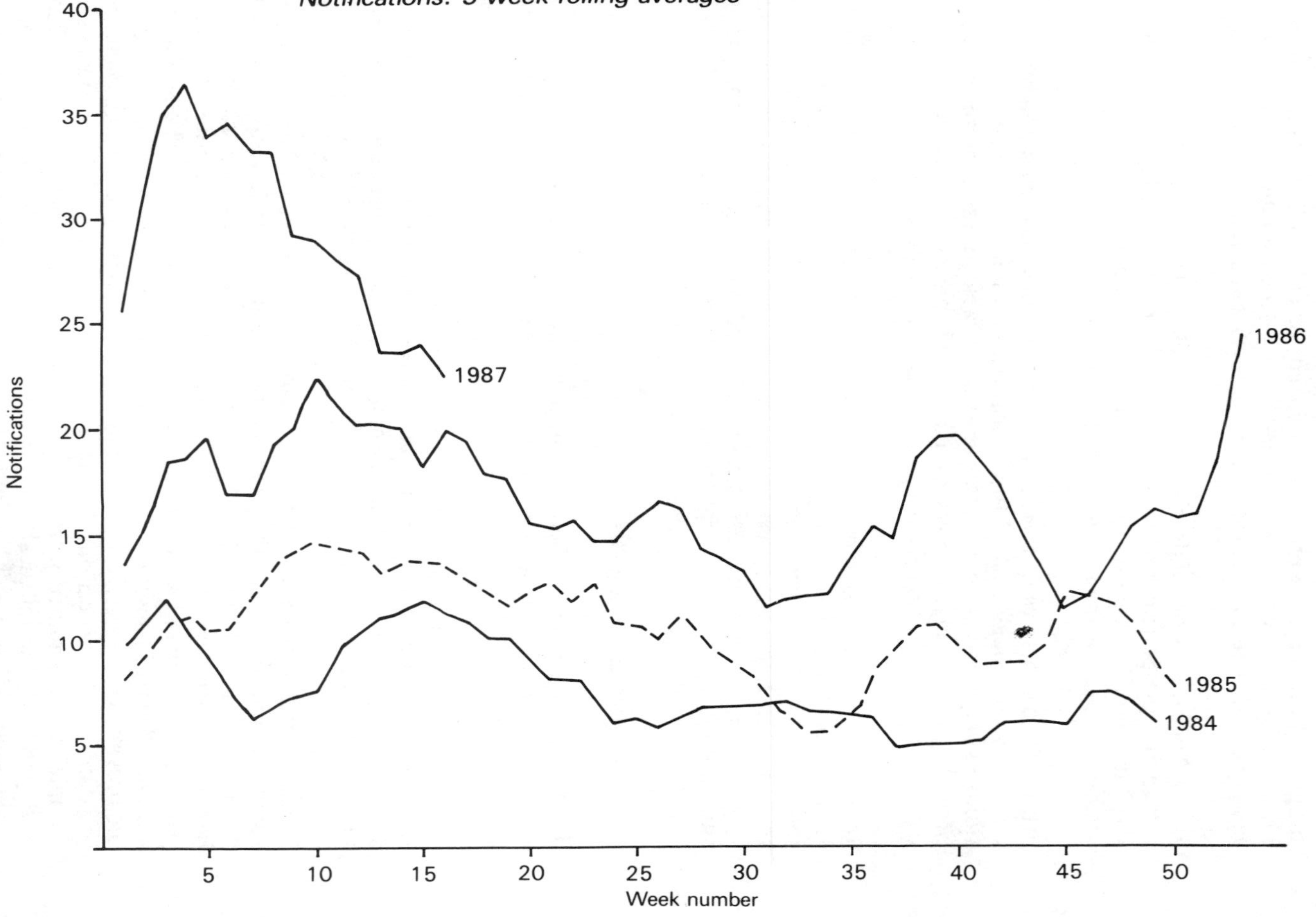

Table 4.7: *Meningococcal infections, 1977–1986, by Group as percentage of grouped organisms*

YEAR	GROUP A	GROUP B	GROUP C
1977	20.1	67.3	16.7
1978	17.4	61.4	17.4
1979	15.1	60.1	18.7
1980	12.1	62.7	20.0
1981	8.8	67.6	20.8
1982	3.9	67.1	26.0
1983	4.2	64.8	26.9
1984	3.9	65.8	27.5
1985	3.0	64.6	30.2
1986	3.3	54.8	40.3

experiencing an outbreak of meningococcal infection from this organism. The distribution of carriers by age-groups shows peak carriage rates in teenagers and young adults with a secondary peak in five to nine-year-old children. This study supports the hypothesis that Group B15 meningococcal infection is associated with low transmissibility but high virulence.

(j) Legionellosis

The *'First Report of the Committee of Inquiry into the outbreak of Legionnaires Disease in Stafford in April 1985'* was published in June 1986[5]. The Committee of Inquiry recommended that a Committee of Experts should be convened to consider biocides used against Legionella. Ministers accepted this recommendation and Dr E A Wright, Director of the Regional Public Health Laboratory, Newcastle upon Tyne, was appointed Chairman of the new Committee. Its terms of reference are 'to consider all aspects of the use of biocides including their efficacy and safety in minimising the risk of multiplication of *Legionella pneumophila* in hospital cooling tower water systems and other water systems in hospitals'. An interim report is expected towards the end of 1987.

In England and Wales, 188 cases (including 22 deaths) — 134 male, 53 female, 1 sex unknown — of Legionnaires disease were reported to the CDSC in 1986 as compared with 211 in 1985. Ninety two of the infections appear to have been acquired abroad. There were 7 clusters of 2 or more cases. Six clusters comprising 13 cases were associated with hotels abroad and there was one outbreak in Gloucester which produced 15 cases.

(k) Tuberculosis

The number of new cases of tuberculosis notified in England and Wales for 1986 was 5,992 and the number of registered deaths (including later effects of the disease) was 733. The trend over the past decade is given in Table 4.8. Examination of age and sex specific mortality data since 1979 reveals a consistent decline among males both for deaths attributed directly to tuberculosis and those attributed to 'late effects of TB'. In contrast, in females aged over 55 years no such consistent decline has occurred, and in some age-groups death rates have risen.

Table 4.8: *Tuberculosis — England and Wales, 1977–1986*

Year	Notified new cases	Deaths
1977	9,490	991
1978	9,673	900
1979	9,269	936
1980	9,144	903
1981	8,128	764
1982†	7,406	750
1983	6,800	699
1984	6,141	753
1985	5,857	773
1986	5,992*	733

† From 1982 onwards notifications associated with chemoprophylaxis are excluded
* Provisional

(l) Malaria

New cases of malaria notified within the UK almost invariably arise in people who have travelled to the UK from known malarious countries. Rarely, usually in the vicinity of an international airport, transmission by escaped infected mosquitoes can occur within the UK. (See *this Report* for 1983, p. 46).

The annual cost of hospital in-patient treatment in England for malaria cases is of the order of £1 million. The number of cases occurring within the UK (1977 to 1986) and reported to the PHLS Malaria Reference Laboratory is shown in Table 4.9. Deaths average 6.5 each year. This table reveals no consistent trend. Figure 4.3 shows the age distribution of those admitted to hospital with malaria in England for the years 1982–84 (HIPE).

Table 4.9: *Malaria reported annually to PHLS Malaria Reference Laboratory (UK), 1977–1986*

Year	Cases	Deaths
1977	1,529	7
1978	1,909	10
1979	2,053	5
1980	1,670	9
1981	1,576	2
1982	1,471	10
1983	1,711	7
1984	1,934	6
1985	2,212	5
1986	2,209	4

Advice on malaria medication is provided for travellers in leaflet SA 35 '*Protect Your Health Abroad*' which is updated annually and distributed by the UK Health Departments to travel agents, vaccination centres and GPs. Travellers are advised to obtain detailed advice on drug prophylaxis from their GPs who may in turn consult the PHLS Malaria Reference Laboratory or other centres that manage infectious and tropical diseases.

Figure 4.3: *Malaria - England, 1982-1984, hospital admissions by age-group*

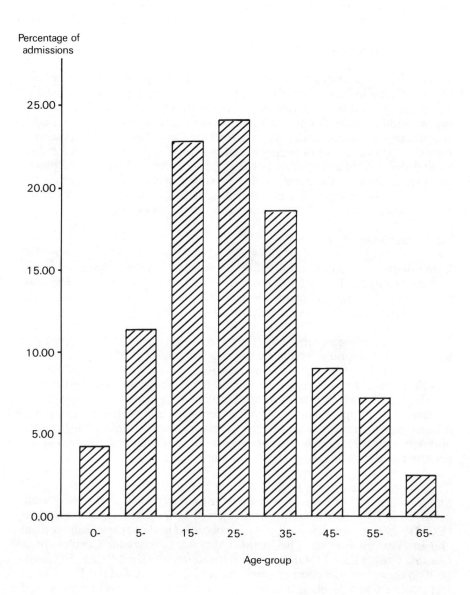

The emergence of resistant strains and the evidence of adverse effects for some of the drugs used require careful assessment and it is not surprising that consensus views on prophylactic regimens are difficult to obtain. The British National Formulary is a ready source of information for medical practitioners and an article on prophylaxis was published in the *Prescribers' Journal* in 1986[6].

(m) Viral haemorrhagic fevers

Much experience of this group of diseases has been gained since a missionary nurse working in Lassa, Nigeria, fell ill in 1969 with an undiagnosed infection. The pathogen was later isolated and named the Lassa virus. Early in 1986 a new memorandum on the Control of Viral Haemorrhagic Fevers was published[7,8]. It contains the recommendations of a Working Party that met over a two year period to update advice originally issued in 1976. Copies of the Memorandum were distributed to all health authorities with a request that it should be passed to all clinicians and others who would be involved in managing any outbreak of the diseases or in caring for patients. A separately printed Summary of the Memorandum was in addition distributed to all doctors in England[9,10].

(n) Lyme disease

Lyme disease is a zoonosis caused by a spirochaete *Borrelia burgdorferi* and transmitted by the bite of a tick (*Ixodes ricinus*). *Borrelia burgdorferi* has also been isolated from small mammals in areas endemic for Lyme disease in the USA. These mammals serve as reservoirs for infection.

Lyme disease is a generalised disorder which is characterised by a spreading annular skin eruption, erythema chronica migrans (ECM). ECM may be followed weeks or months later by arthritis, neurological and cardiological manifestations. Patients experience recurrent disabling attacks of arthritis of the large joints which may become chronic and destructive. They may also present with chronic meningitis, with encephalitis and peripheral motor and sensory neuropathy or radiculopathy. Cardiac conduction defects, myocarditis and pericarditis also occur. Past or current infections can be diagnosed by the presence of circulating antibodies to the spirochaete.

The name of the disease is derived from Lyme, Connecticut in the United States, where an outbreak of juvenile arthritis associated with the spirochaete occurred in 1985. Subsequently many infected patients developed skin lesions (ECM)[11]. Since then sporadic cases have occurred in East Anglia and Scotland and in Western Europe. The British Laboratory Reference Centres are at Charing Cross Hospital and the Leptospira Reference Unit, PHLS, Hertford. In 1986 there were 68 cases of Lyme diseases in the UK and the Republic of Ireland[12]. ECM was observed in 41 patients and 8 of them had associated neurological disease. The neurological disease without preceding skin lesion occurred in 13 further patients. Myocarditis was present in 1 patient. In 2 areas deer were found to be infected by *Borrelia burgdorferi* and 68% of 45 deer sera tested had significant antibody against *B. burgdorferi*. Early treatment with tetracycline or penicillin will abort the disease.

Several review articles on Lyme disease dealing with the ecology of ticks and with the epidimeology and laboratory diagnosis of the infection were published in the July 1987 issue of the PHLS *Microbiology Digest*.

(o) Ovine abortion

During 1986 veterinary and farming journals publicised the association between *Chlamydia psittaci* and human abortion[13,14]. Obstetricians working in agricultural areas should also be aware of this relatively uncommon but potentially serious problem. In sheep, the organism *Chlamydia psittaci* causes abortion, stillbirth and sickly lambs. A small number of cases in which *Chlamydia psittaci* has been the cause of abortion in pregnant women attending infective ewes during the lambing season have now been documented. Some of the women were severely ill with intravascular coagulation, acute renal failure and pulmonary oedema. Pregnant women who are attending lambing ewes should be informed about the dangers of *Chlamydia psittaci*, particularly when epidemics among their flocks are known. Three cases were reported in England in the Spring of 1986.

In December MAFF issued a Press Release about the risks of the disease to pregnant women[15]. The veterinary profession, the Agricultural Development and Advisory Service and the Health and Safety Executive also provide advice.

(p) Microbiology of food/Food poisoning

Notifications and cases ascertained by other means reported to the OPCS by Medical Officers for Environmental Health (MOsEH) in England and Wales are included in weekly, quarterly and annual OPCS publications. Table 4.10

Table 4.10: *Food poisoning cases in England 1982–6 corrected notifications to OPCS*

	Year	Formally notified	Ascertained by other means	Total
Presumed contracted abroad	1982	866	421	1,287
	1983	1,006	559	1,605
	1984	1,062	685	1,747
	1985	1,022	653	1,675
	1986	1,352	837	2,189
Presumed contracted in GB	1982	7,022	3,085	10,107
	1983	8,651	3,503	12,454
	1984	9,607	5,403	15,010
	1985	8,862	4,168	13,030
	1986	11,239	4,858	16,097
Not known where contracted	1982	1,468	714	2,182
	1983	1,954	1,008	2,962
	1984	1,776	1,211	2,987
	1985	2,078	1,101	3,179
	1986	2,673	1,565	4,238
Totals	1982	9,356	4,220	13,576
	1983	11,611	5,410	17,021
	1984	12,445	7,299	19,744
	1985	11,962	5,922	17,884
	1986	15,264	7,260	22,524

Foot-Note: There were 53 reporting weeks in 1986.

gives extracts, relating to England only from the OPCS collations for 5 years 1982–6. The numbers of notifications and reports have increased steadily throughout the period and in 1986 outbreaks were the highest on record. Salmonellosis and campylobacter enteritis continue to be the most important foodborne infections in England. Provisional data from CDSC for 1986 show an increase of both laboratory identifications of Salmonellas to almost 15,000 and laboratory reports of campylobacter enteritis to around 24,500.

(i) Contamination of milk powder products
In December 1985 a food company withdrew its baby food mix powder products after an epidemiological investigation proved that *Salmonella ealing* contamination in the powder was causing illness in babies. The withdrawal operation, subsequent investigation and cleaning operation at the factory affected its viability and the parent company sold it. The new parent company immediately introduced procedures and controls which have led to the safe resumption of production and sale of baby food powders.

Following this experience major UK manufacturers of milk powder products reviewed their manufacturing procedures and quality controls and increased sampling surveillance of the factory environments and products. Mainly as a result of this increased surveillance there were 3 occasions in 1986 when manufacturers isolated Salmonella in product powders. In the detailed factory investigations which took place as a result of these findings Salmonellas were also discovered in the environments of the 3 factories concerned.

Withdrawals and detailed screening of various powder products were carried out with detailed factory cleaning and disinfection of surfaces and equipment. It was not possible to establish precisely how the milk powder became contaminated. Some form of post-process contamination was most likely because temperatures achieved during pasteurisation, evaporation and spray drying procedures will eliminate pathogenic organisms (including Salmonella) in the incoming raw milk.

The presence of Salmonella may be explained in several ways. Incoming raw milk may contain Salmonella which, while being handled in the factory prior to heat processing, contaminates surfaces, worker's clothing or equipment. This contamination may later be transferred to the area of the spray drier. Moisture must be eliminated from this environment because Salmonella accompanied by moisture and appropriate temperature can lead to the contamination of the internal surfaces of the drier. Salmonella may then contaminate milk powder during the final stages of the manufacturing process. It is also possible that birds carrying Salmonella may have entered the factories. Bird droppings were considered to be the source of a Salmonella contamination of a milk powder plant in Australia in 1977. The droppings on the roof led to contamination of the spray dry area. Another secondary hazard arises from animal faeces adhering to tanker tyres.

Following these experiences the Department, together with MAFF and the PHLS, met with the Association of British Preserved Milk Manufacturers to draw up guidelines for good hygienic practice in the manufacture of milk powders. A second draft of these guidelines prepared by the Association was under consideration at the end of 1986. They became available in 1987.

(ii) Milk

In March 1986 an outbreak of *Salmonella braenderup* in Cambridge involved 26 primary cases and several asymptomatic excreters. Pasteurised milk was identified as the vehicle of infection. A further 5 excreters of the salmonella were identified on a farm which supplied raw milk to the dairy associated with the outbreak. Organisms were found in bulk milk and dairy equipment at the dairy. The pasteurised milk may have been contaminated in the dairy by mixing with raw milk. The operational procedures in the plant were reviewed.

Salmonellosis from drinking raw cow's milk appears to be increasing, but infection due to pasteurised milk is exceptional. Milkborne disease in England and Wales between 1938 and 1982 was reviewed[16]. During this period there were 179 outbreaks of milkborne salmonellosis (3,818 cases and 7 deaths). Only one of them was associated with pasteurised milk. Outbreaks increased during the period under study — 10 between 1941 and 1950, 25 between 1951 and 1960, 50 between 1961 and 1970, 73 between 1971 and 1980 and 52 in the 4 years 1981–1984. The causative serotypes changed. Outbreaks due to *S. typhimurium* increased, whereas those due to *S. dublin* decreased during the 1970s. These changes have been attributed to changes in dairy practice such as increase in the size of herds, pipe-line milking and bulk collection of milk[17] as has been seen in Scotland. Compulsory pasteurisation would greatly reduce milkborne salmonellosis. However, recent outbreaks caused by dried and pasteurised milk emphasise that high standards of hygiene and maintenance in pasteurisation and milk drying plants are very important.

(iii) Salmonella contamination of creamed coconut

Late in 1986 a national distributor of confectionery and coconut products isolated a Salmonella in creamed coconut supplied by a small manufacturer in the West Midlands. The coconut is made into a paste and spread on to the surface of meals prepared in Indian restaurants. Detailed examination revealed several isolations of Salmonella. The Division of Enteric Pathogens (PHLS) confirmed 3 serotypes among the distributed products.

Sri Lankan desiccated coconut was found to be contaminated. Coconut supplied by brokers and scrapings of desiccated coconut taken from an emulsifier in the manufacturing plant were both affected.

A total of 5½ tonnes of packaged creamed coconut returned to the manufacturer and half of the Sri Lankan desiccated coconut were destroyed and the loss to the manufacturer was about £25,000. The manufacturing equipment was stripped and disinfected. A sample run using Ivory Coast desiccated coconut then proved negative for salmonella.

The incident was referred to the Sri Lankan High Commission who took the matter up with the Coconut Development Authority in Sri Lanka where the reasons for the contaminated import were investigated early in 1987.

No illness from the consumption of the desiccated creamed coconut was reported in the UK.

(iv) Salmonella in imported liquid whole egg

Two workers in a bakery in the North East of England became ill with *Salmonella enteritidis* after handling liquid egg used for glazing confectionery products. A total of 120 employees at the bakery were screened. Six reported gastro-intestinal symptoms but only 2 were positive the *Salmonella enteritidis*. They were thought to have become infected as a result of handling the liquid whole egg.

The liquid egg came from an importer in the North East who obtained it from Belgium for processing and despatch from a liquid egg processing plant. The consignment at the bakery had been imported as a pasteurised product and had been given no further treatment prior to despatch.

The Liquid Egg (Pasteurisation) Regulations 1963 require imports of liquid whole egg to be pasteurised before or on arrival in the UK. The failure to pasteurise the product had been the cause of illness in the bakery workers and the importer seemed to have breached the Regulations.

All liquid egg stock at the bakery was returned for further pasteurisation and intensive sampling. Imported products are now being processed as a routine by the importer/processor. The Belgian Food Inspection Service was contacted and action was taken at the premises of the Belgian exporting plant.

The bakery produced a number of products in which liquid egg is used as an ingredient or as a glaze. Survival of low levels of Salmonellae after bakery processing is possible. The whole question of both liquid egg and eggs in shell being used in bakery and the survival of Salmonellae during the heat processing is being investigated.

(v) Shellfish
Twelve (12) incidents of gastro-enteritis associated with molluscan shellfish, particularly cockles, occurred during the 1986 pre-Christmas period; 250 persons were ill. Small round structured viruses and parvoviruses were found in stool specimens of affected persons and on one occasion pathogens were isolated from the shellfish samples. Outbreaks were similar to those reported in the winter of 1985/86 when there were 62 incidents affecting over 500 people.

The cockles originated from Leigh-on-Sea. Early in 1987 urgent action has been taken in the following areas:

(i)   Upgrading the manufacturing processes in the Leigh cockle sheds.

(ii)   A voluntary ban was applied to fishing cockles from known polluted estuarial water areas;

(iii)   Improvement in labelling and identification of products; and

(iv)   The Leigh cockle fishmen will meet regularly with the City of London Port Health staff and the Southend Borough Environmental Health staff to review procedures.

(vi) Gastro-enteritis on a cruise ship

During the months of May to June 1986 a cruise ship had outbreaks of gastro-enteritis on 7 successive cruises. Initially the causative organism was considered to be an enterotoxigenic strain of *Escherichia Coli* but later investigations and isolations from faecal specimens of affected passengers revealed a small round Norwalk-like virus. It was thought to be associated with the ship's water supply. The victims developed a mild febrile illness with vomiting and diarrhoea which lasted about 24 hours and appeared on the 7th or 8th day of the cruises. Intensive improvements in sanitation procedures included increasing chlorine levels of the water supply, improved general hygiene in the galleys, and throughout the ship. Combined with the use of bottled drinking water these measures controlled the outbreak.

(q) Vaccination and immunisation

Table 4.11 shows the number and the percentage of children completing primary courses of vaccination over the last 10 years. The target level for immunisation against measles, whooping cough, diphtheria, tetanus, poliomyelitis and rubella is 90%. There has been an improvement in recent years and in 1985 86% of schoolgirls were vaccinated against rubella by the age of 14 years. However much greater increase in uptake of pertussis vaccine is desirable.

Table 4.11: *Numbers (in thousands) of children aged 16 and under completing primary course of vaccination (with the percentage of eligible children vaccinated before three years of age shown in parenthesis, but for BCG this percentage is the estimated school population age 13 years), England 1975–1985*

Year	Diptheria	Tetanus	Polio	Whooping cough	Measles	BCG
1975	479.0 (74)	499.2 (74)	481.5 (74)	247.9 (60)	310.2 (47)	522.5 (70)
1976	487.8 (75)	510.2 (75)	495.6 (75)	240.6 (38)	323.7 (47)	564.4 (74)
1977	490.0 (78)	513.1 (78)	515.6 (78)	191.9 (40)	304.9 (50)	590.1 (76)
1978	506.0 (78)	524.4 (79)	518.8 (78)	199.4 (31)	302.1 (48)	576.6 (73)
1979	528.6 (80)	543.7 (80)	533.6 (80)	205.3 (35)	331.7 (51)	563.9 (73)
1980	545.9 (81)	560.2 (81)	549.7 (81)	285.6 (41)	351.6 (53)	617.9 (81)
1981	552.2 (83)	564.4 (83)	554.5 (82)	320.5 (46)	368.5 (55)	575.1 (78)
1982	558.1 (84)	572.7 (84)	562.8 (84)	584.8 (53)	390.7 (58)	547.1 (75)
1983	528.5 (84)	538.3 (84)	531.5 (84)	406.8 (59)	392.9 (60)	538.1 (76)
1984	532.1 (84)	540.2 (84)	534.0 (84)	391.7 (65)	435.6 (63)	507.9 (71)
1985	544.4 (85)	551.6 (85)	548.9 (85)	414.2 (65)	473.8 (68)	518.7 (72)*

* Provisional figure

References

[1] Miller C L, Miller E, Waight P A. Rubella susceptibility and the continuing risk of infection in pregnancy. *Br Med J* 198; **294:** 1277–8.

[2] Public Health Laboratory Service Communicable Disease Surveillance Centre. Communicable disease report: October to December 1986. *Community Med* 1987; **9:** 176–81.

[3] Department of Health and Social Security. *Influenze.* London: Department of Health and Social Security, 1987; DHSS circular CMO(86)15.

[4] Department of Health and Social Security. *Influenza.* London: Department of Health and Social Security, 1987; DHSS circular CMO(87)2.

[5] Department of Health and Social Security. *First report of the Committee of Inquiry into the Outbreak of Legionnaires Disease in Stafford in April 1985.* Department of Health and Social Security, 1986, London: HMSO, 1986.

[6] Walker E. Malaria prophylaxis. *Prescribers' Journal* 1986; **26:** 39/45.

[7] Department of Health and Social Security. *Memorandum on the control of viral haemorrhagic fevers.* London: Department of Health and Social Security, 1986; DHSS circular CMO(86)3.

[8] Department of Health and Social Security and the Welsh Office. *Memorandum on the control of viral haemorrhagic fevers*, 1986; London: HMSO.

[9] Department of Health and Social Security. *Summary of the memorandum on the control of viral haemorrhagic fevers*. London: Department of Health and Social Security, 1986. DHSS circular CMO(86)4.

[10] Department of Health and Social Security and the Welsh Office. *Summary of the memorandum on the control of viral haemorrhagic fevers*. London: Department of Health and Social Security, 1986.

[11] Parke A. From new to old England: The progress of Lyme disease. *Br Med J* 1987; **294:** 525–6.

[12] Muhleman M F, Wright D J M. Emerging pattern of Lyme disease in the United Kingdom and Irish Republic. *Lancet* 1987; **i:** 260–2.

[13] Buxton D. Potential danger to pregnant women of *Chlamydia psittaci* from sheep. *Vet Rec* 1986; **118:** 510–1.

[14] Eddy R G, Martin W B. Pregnant women and chlamydia infection (letter). *Vet Rec* 1986; **118:** 519.

[15] Ministry of Agriculture, Fisheries and Food. *Joint announcement by the Ministry of Agriculture, Fisheries and Food and the Department of Health and Social Security: enzootic abortion in ewes: hazard to pregnant women at lambing time.* London: MAFF, 1986; MAFF press release 9 December 1986.

[16] Galbraith N S, Pusey J J. Milkborne infectious diseases in England and Wales 1938–1982. In: Freed D L J, ed. *Health hazards of milk.* London: Bailliere Tindall, 1984; 27–59.

[17] Barrett N J. Communicable disease associated with milk and dairy products in England and Wales: 1983–1984. *J Infect* 1986; **12:** 265–72.

(r) Sexually transmitted disease

Clinics in England reported 605,306 (332,840 male and 272,466 female) new cases in 1985 (Tables 4.12 and 4.13). This represents an increase of 6.2% over 1984, being greater in females (9%) than in males (4%). The majority of the increase in case-load was attributable to attendances for non-specific genital infection (10,172 additional cases) and for diseases classified as 'other conditions', both those requiring and not requiring treatment (9,105 and 9,211 additional cases respectively). A large rise also occurred in attendance for genital warts, resulting in an increase of 18% over 1984.

The problems produced by the human immunodeficiency virus (HIV) influenced the work in clinics markedly. Clinics in London continued to treat increasing numbers of cases of AIDS and HIV infections, and smaller numbers of cases attended clinics elsewhere in England. The availability of tests for HIV antibody resulted in diagnosis of individuals with asymptomatic infection. These data have been presented elsewhere in this report.

Over the years clinics have adapted to increasing numbers of patients by increasing their management efficiency. However, patients with AIDS/HIV infection or concerned about such infection, require more time than those with other sexually transmitted diseases. This greatly adds to the already increasing workload being undertaken by the clinics.

(i) Gonorrhoea

A steady decline in the reported incidence of gonorrhoea masks important differences in secular trends at different ages. Age-specific data are presented in Figures 4.4 and 4.5 and illustrate how in recent years the decline in disease rate has, in both sexes, been greatest at older ages, particularly in those aged 35–44 years and to a lesser extent those aged 25–34 years. Gonorrhoea infection rates provide important clues to current patterns of sexual behaviour and the steepening in the rate of decline apparent from 1982 in males aged over 35 years, may represent a change in behaviour among homosexual men following publicity concerning the risk of AIDS infection. Of concern though is the lack of recent decline in males and females aged 16–19 years who have a high underlying disease rate. In fact, there was a small rise in disease rate in this age-group in both sexes in 1985. Monitoring of such age-specific trends will be a matter of considerable importance in the years to come.

Isolates of β-lactamase-producing totally penicillin-resistant *Neisseria gonorrhoea* fell for the second consecutive year. This contrasts with the situation in many other countries where these isolates are either increasing or maintaining a high incidence.

(ii) Syphilis

Between 1984 and 1985 there was a substantial fall in the total number of new cases of syphilis attending GUM clinics (Table 4.12). This mainly reflected a 35% decline in the incidence of primary and secondary syphilis. Figures 4.6 and 4.7 present age-specific time trends for these forms of the disease. In women, although there are inconsistencies, particularly at older ages where numbers of cases are few, a general pattern of decline is apparent in all age-groups. A more

77

Table 4.12: *Cases of syphilis and gonorrhoea reported by NHS GUM clinics in England for the year ended 31 December 1985 with the figures for the year ended 31 December 1984 in parentheses*

	Total		Male		Female	
Syphilis						
Early	1,229	(1,702)	1,032	(1,475)	197	(227)
Primary and secondary only	691	(1,032)	625	(923)	66	(109)
Late	1,107	(1,167)	759	(815)	348	(325)
Congenital	68	(64)	28	(25)	40	(39)
Gonorrhoea						
All forms	46,314	(47,662)	28,759	(29,791)	17,555	(17,871)
Post-pubertal gonorrhoea						
All ages	46,294	(47,643)	28,751	(29,789)	17,543	(17,854)
Under 16 years	317	(360)	73	(94)	244	(266)
16–19 years	10,286	(10,295)	4,438	(4,398)	5,848	(5,897)
20–24 years	18,370	(18,285)	11,363	(11,188)	7,007	(7,097)
25–34 years	12,830	(13,343)	9,231	(9,709)	3,559	(3,634)
35–44 years	3,299	(3,952)	2,615	(3,187)	584	(765)
45 years and over	1,192	(1,408)	1,031	(1,213)	161	(195)

Table 4.13: *Other sexually transmitted diseases reported in England in the year ended 31 December 1985 with the figures for 31 December 1984 in parentheses*

	Total		Male		Female	
Chancroid	61	(40)	48	(31)	13	(9)
Lymphogranuloma venereum	30	(30)	23	(23)	7	(7)
Granuloma inguinale	17	(19)	15	(15)	2	(4)
Non-specific genital infection (NSGI)	149,524	(139,352)	103,198	(99,497)	46,326	(39,855)
NSGI with arthritis	487	(428)	459	(407)	28	(21)
Trichomoniasis	15,381	(16,751)	1,077	(1,211)	14,304	(15,540)
Candidiasis	60,517	(59,688)	11,853	(12,133)	48,664	(47,535)
Scabies	2,015	(2,043)	1,644	(1,693)	351	(350)
Pediculosis pubis	9,859	(10,183)	6,817	(7,042)	3,042	(3,141)
Genital herpes	18,935	(18,301)	10,025	(9,663)	8,910	(8,638)
Genital warts	52,177	(44,050)	31,250	(26,899)	20,927	(17,151)
Genital molluscum	2,195	(1,928)	1,374	(1,230)	821	(698)
Other treponemal diseases	592	(658)	384	(425)	208	(233)
Other conditions requiring treatment in a centre	109,318	(100,213)	49,079	(47,817)	60,239	(52,396)
Other conditions not requiring treatment in a centre	130,162	(120,951)	82,242)	(76,789)	47,920	(44,162)
Other conditions referred elsewhere	5,318	(4,718)	2,754	(2,502)	2,564	(2,216)
Overall Total	605,306					

Figure 4.4: *New cases of post-pubertal gonorrhoea, males, age specific rates per 100,000 population, England 1976-1985*

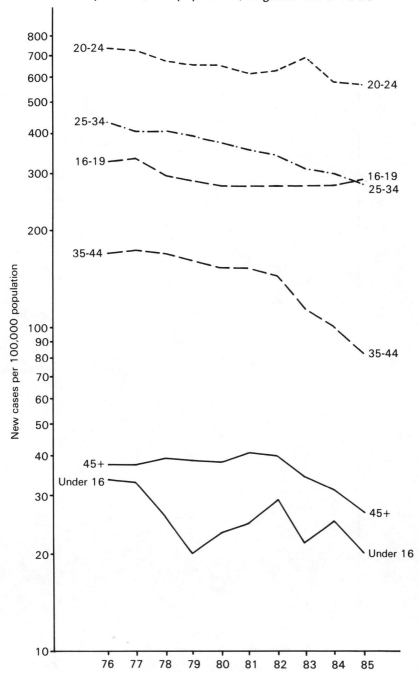

Note: *Population aged 45 to 59 is used to calculate rates at ages of 45 and over*

Figure 4.5: *New cases of post-pubertal gonorrhoea, females, age specific rates per 100,000 population, England 1976-1985*

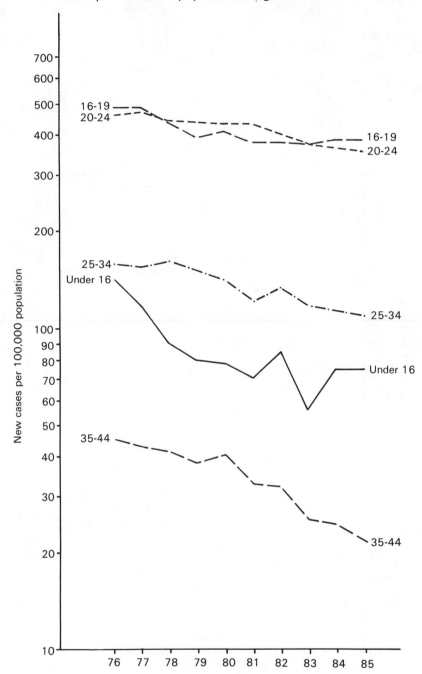

Note: *Population aged 45 to 59 is used to calculate rates at ages of 45 and over*

consistent decline has also occurred in males although above the age of 35 years the decline did not start until the early 1980s. In the three older age-groups the decline in males was particularly pronounced in 1985, perhaps again reflecting changes in sexual behaviour. In the 16–19 age-group, in contrast to gonorrhoea, there has been a marked decline in syphilis between 1976 and the present.

Regional variations occur, and the fall in both syphilis and gonorrhoea has been more marked in the Thames region than elsewhere. Some forms of syphilis have shown small rises in 1985, as in early latent syphilis in females where numbers of new cases rose from 118 in 1984 to 131 in 1985, the rate of new cases now approaching the 1975 level. This emphasises the need to maintain control measures such as ante-natal screening as mentioned in *this Report* in 1985 (page 60). Although there was a small rise in reported cases of congenital syphilis in 1985, no case of early congenital disease was reported.

(iii) Genital warts

The number of new cases presenting with genital warts increased in 1985, reflecting the consistent rise in reported incidence of this disease over the last few years (Figure 4.8) Genital warts now account for almost 9% of the total of new cases seen at GUM clinics. Media attention to the association between genital warts, cervical dyskaryosis and carcinoma has made the public more aware of the condition. More patients may therefore be attending clinics for examination and treatment. During the year, the limitations of cervical smears as a screening technique was further exposed, and this has led to increasing pressure on the colposcopic service within clinics.

(iv) Genital herpes simplex

A small rise in new cases of genital herpes occurred in 1985 continuing the trend of the last 10 years (Figure 4.8). The rise in both sexes was however less than in recent years. Since 1975 reported incidence of disease has risen more sharply in females than males, and female rates are now only slightly less than male rates.

(v) Non-specific genital infection

In 1985 new cases of non-specific genital infection rose to 149,524 and now account for almost one quarter of all new cases attending clinics. Examination of time trends (Figure 4.8) reveals a steady but slow rise in male incidence rates, in contrast to a steeper rise present in women. In 1985 the annual increase was 16% in females compared to 3% in males. In previous reports it was suggested that similar increases may have been due to increased availability of investigations for *Chlamydia trachomatis*. This more dramatic increase may be an indication of greater public awareness of pelvic inflammatory disease and increased contact tracing among female partners of infected males.

(vi) Trichomoniasis and candidiasis

These diseases show differing trends. A steady fall in new cases of trichomoniasis has occurred in both sexes since 1980. The decline has continued in 1985 with a 12% fall in males and a 9% fall in females. Candidiasis rose steadily in both sexes over the same period until 1985, when the rise continued in females, but there was a small fall in males.

Figure 4.6: *New cases of primary and secondary syphilis, males 1976-1985, age specific rates per 100,000 population, England*

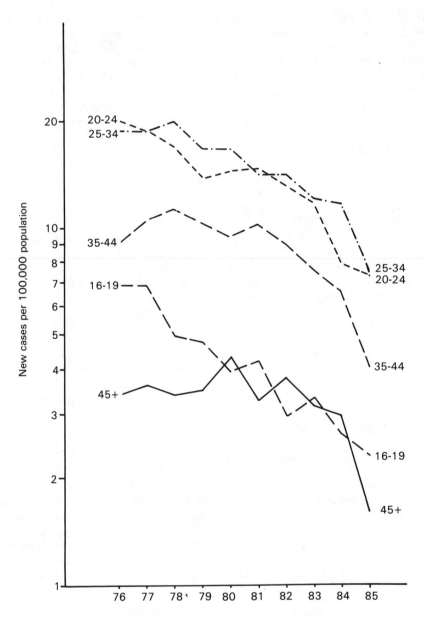

Note: *Population aged 45 to 59 is used to calculate rates at ages of 45 and over.*

Figure 4.7: *New cases of primary and secondary syphilis, females, 1976-1985, Age specific rates per 100,000 population, England*

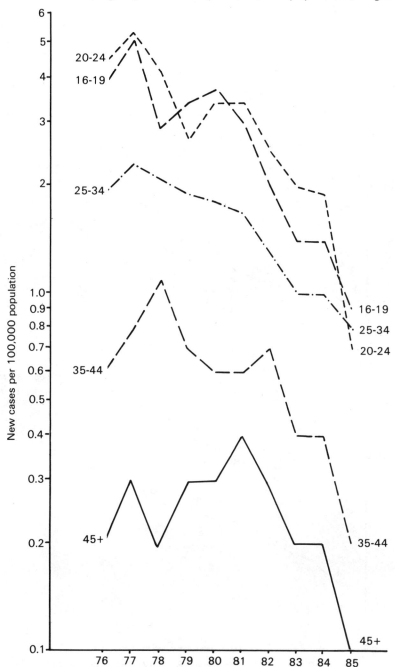

Note: *The population aged 45 to 59 is used to calculate rates of 45 and over.*

Figure 4.8: *New cases of selected diseases, males and females, 1975-85, rates per 100,000 population, England*

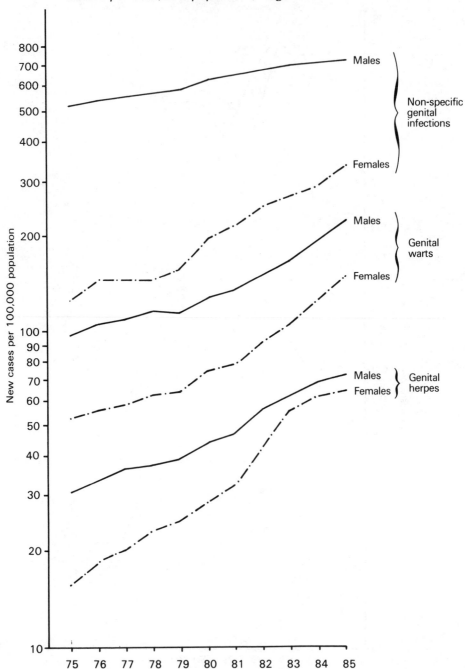

(vii) Other conditions

Other conditions requiring treatment continued to show the upward trend apparent for the previous decade. The 1984/5 rise in reported incidence in females (14%) was considerably greater than that in males (2%). The latter figure includes cases of HIV infection. In females the rise may reflect more widespread recognition of anaerobic or bacterial vaginosis. Some clinic medical staff are concerned about the increasing number of conditions grouped under this heading as important trends may be concealed.

As part of the Körner review, the content of the form SBH 60 is to be revised from 1 April 1988, to take account of some of the criticisms which have been raised. For example, chlamydia, vaginosis, HIV, hepatitis and some other conditions will be separately identified to try to reduce the numbers of cases recorded under the NSGI and 'Other conditions' headings. We will be separately identifying homosexually acquired infections and asking for a count of first-ever presentations of some recurrent conditions eg herpes, to attempt to get an estimate of the spread throughout the population.

(viii) Statistical Bulletin on STD

Further information on rates of new cases seen at NHS genito-urinary clinics can be obtained from the Statistical Bulletin on Sexually Transmitted Diseases. This is obtainable from Information Division (DHSS), Cannons Park, Government Buildings, Honeypot Lane, Stanmore HAY IAY — Price £1.00.

5. PRIMARY HEALTH CARE

This report for 1985 (p. 65) referred to the steady progress in primary health care in recent years with the improvement of premises, the employment of a wider range of staff and the development of new patterns of care, particularly for the elderly and people with mental illness and mental handicap. Simultaneously research, often undertaken in academic units, has increased knowledge about the activities in general practice and the opportunities which exist. The work of the Royal College of General Practitioners (RCGP) Research Unit based in Birmingham on the National Morbidity Surveys which are carried out in census years and cover roughly 300,000 patients and over 100 GPs, has shown how very slowly the nature of patients' complaints change although the nature of the GP's care may be different. The main categories of disease remain the same although practitioners are initiating more preventive procedures than they used to. Studies of workload, including the survey carried out jointly by the DHSS and the General Medical Services Committee (GMSC) in 1985/6 and other surveys from Canterbury and Manchester[1,2] revealed more about the pattern of a doctor's working day, the contact rates, and how these relate to types of area and list size. The Canterbury work supports the view that doctors differ in their interests, some being more interested in minor surgery, others in prevention and some with a particular concern for matters like the health problems of women. Workers in York identified other differences, for example groups of young doctors who invest highly in their practices often at a cost of their personal income, and other older doctors who tend to be more traditional in their approach but who show a greater willingness to undertake home visiting. It is sometimes stated that while the total costs of the family practitioner service are considerable, what GPs actually do is not known. That is only partly true; ignorance mainly concerns the way they do it, their style and the quality of their care. Like most aspects of the NHS general practice exhibits wide variations in performance.

The Department commissioned a project in the Northern Region in 1982 to see if GPs could improve their performance by working together in small groups to draw up explicit standards for care. Ten groups of trainers from 65 practices, working with the Department of Child Health and the Health Care Research Unit, have been setting clinical standards for 5 common childhood illnesses.

Scrutiny of medical records and interviews with parents are being used to test whether standard setting changes clinical conduct and improves the welfare of the children.

Other research work is helping to define the information required for good practice. Criteria for clinical records have been proposed. An increasing number of doctors are using microcomputers and this helps to define what should be recorded to ensure that patients receive the services they need, particularly in the field of preventive medicine and anticipatory health care. Some doctors keep computer held summaries of patients' past medical histories. With the increase in community care for the elderly and people with mental illness, and the many different disciplines involved effective communication and good records are essential. The Department is supporting a project in Wales using a 'smart card', which resembles a credit card but contains a memory and sometimes a minute processor. This allows the transfer of information between GPs and pharmacists and enables the use of technology in treatment to be explored. Such systems are likely to have an increasing impact on clinical care.

Prescribing has also been a subject of interest because it is a useful model for methods of improving the quality of care. Research has explored the acceptability of feeding back prescribing information; when the information is concise and well presented it is welcomed.

This encouraged a study of the effectiveness of information to see whether or not GPs alter their prescribing habits if given data about their own performance and an opportunity to discuss them with other practitioners. Almost certainly this resulted in more thoughtful prescribing, and there were demonstrable reductions in the frequency and cost per item of prescribing once GPs were encouraged to discuss their routines with colleagues. A follow-up study of the same doctors 2 years later showed that most of the effects had worn off — though an increase in generic prescribing persisted. Continuing interest seems necessary to bring about lasting change. There has been an increase in the number of doctors seeking information about their own prescribing, in many cases so that they can discuss it with colleagues. There is also a small but growing interest in the development of local formularies. These initiatives by the medical profession itself are warmly welcomed.

Some developments have involved action research. The Norfolk Health Authority has developed a scheme which provides additional support to GPs, by attaching community dieticians, physiotherapists and psychiatric nurses to groups of practices. This is a welcome and practical example of a new way of organising primary health care. The King's Fund has also been looking at new approaches in the context of its London Programme and at the use of development workers. Good premises make it possible for the various disciplines to work with each other to the benefit of the patient. The work of the Medical Architecture Research Unit demonstrates how older premises can be converted to provide high quality accommodation for primary health care teams, particularly in London. The closeness of team working has been shown to correlate with the ability to house staff under the same roof, which remains a problem in some inner cities.

The Primary Health Care Discussion Document

In spite of this increasing knowledge and the progressive development in primary health care in recent years the government believed that good though the services were, they could be better still.

The introduction to the annual report for 1985 noted the publication in April 1986 of the Primary Health Care Discussion Document (CMND 9771)[3]. Simultaneously the Cumberlege Report on Community Nursing Services was published[4]. During the consultation period Ministers chaired 10 public meetings in various parts of the country on the proposals in these documents and at the end of the year Ministers began to consider the comments received.

The government stated, in publishing the Primary Health Care Discussion Document, that it aims were to improve primary health care services by making them more responsive to the needs of patients, raising standards of care, emphasising the promotion of good health and the prevention of illness, and ensuring that the taxpayer received value for money. Were pharmacists being used to best advantage? Was the full potential of nurses being realised? Could family doctors be helped to make more effective use of their particular skills and knowledge?

Among other proposals the discussion document suggested the introduction of allowances to encourage and reward higher standards of performance, that the proportion of a doctor's pay which was related to the number of patients on his list should be greater, that there should be a compulsory retirement age for GPs, and '24 hour retirement' should be phased out. The government wished to see more detailed information about practices made more widely available, improvements to the complaints procedures and simplification of the system of changing doctors. A greater emphasis on primary care in medical education, and on prevention, was proposed with an increasing role for family doctors in the medical aspects of surveillance of children under school age.

The foreword of the Cumberlege Report said that nurses were at their most effective when they and GPs worked together as an active primary health care team delivering comprehensive care to the consumer.

Its main proposals were that community nursing services should be planned, organised and provided on a neighbourhood basis of 10–25,000, that more and better use could be made of nursing skills, that the effectiveness of primary health care teams needed to be improved and that consumer groups should have a stronger voice.

Topics for discussion

The trend to the organisation of health care services on a local basis is an important development which predates the Cumberlege Report. For a number of years many local authorities have been organising and delivering services like housing from a locally based unit rather than from a central and distant office. The experience has been that housing and social services are more accessible at the neighbourhood centres and that problems are put right more quickly and sensitively. In the health service this concept is also being explored, partly because of the need to provide care for the mentally ill and the mentally handicapped in the community rather than distant hospitals. GPs have, of course, always worked within and for a local population. Now that health authorities and local authorities are considering organistion on a similar basis there is a new opportunity to integrate services for the benefit of the patient.

Quality has become a major national issue both in public services and in industry. Indeed it is one of the hallmarks of a profession that it sets its standards and monitors performance and the establishment of the General Medical Council in 1858 was symbolic of this. From the viewpoint of the public health, quality is one of the most important issues in primary care, and this is recognised both by the GMSC and the RCGP. Much of the 1966 Charter was based upon the relationship between remuneration and the facilities provided. The Charter was largely about the structural features which made for quality in the general medical services.

Government can encourage changes but there is a limit to its ability directly to improve the standard of care provided to individual patients. As independent contractors, GPs bear, both individually and as members of a profession, the main responsibility in this field. During the last 20 years it has become accepted practice for the practices to which vocational trainees are attached to be examined. The Joint Committee on Professional Training for General Practice identifies standards for such practices and indirectly this influences many others. The GMSC of the BMA has, from the mid-sixties onwards, argued that there should be a relationship between the payments system and the work undertaken by GPs. In 1979 a special conference of Local Medical Committees (LMCs) approved the principle of clinical audit of professional standards in general practice. The 'Quality Initiative' of the RCGP launched in 1985, took this a stage further, suggesting that there was support in the profession for the principle of linking performance review with a financial incentive. Since then many local projects have started, often based on peer review of the process by which care is delivered. Individual doctors and nurses are trying out new ideas and are increasingly providing information for leaflets for their patients. Some are producing annual practice reports for LMCs, colleagues or patients to explain what they are trying to achieve. Initiatives in this field include the launching of the King's Fund's Quality Assurance Project.

Disbursing as it does massive sums of public money on health services, the government is inevitably concerned with the quality of services and the value obtained. In the Primary Health Care Discussion Document it proposed the explicit financial recognition of high professional standards of practice. In the USA it has been customary for years for doctors to work within a framework of performance review. But direct linkage of pay with quality assessment and assurance is uncommon. The British proposal would therefore have broken new ground and there were inevitably questions about how such assessments could be fair; and the reasons for the rejection of awards in 1966 were re-iterated in 1986 during the consultation period. While performance related pay has been introduced elsewhere in the NHS, for example for senior managers of regional and district health authorities, the problems in medicine are certainly complex and require a consideration of clinical outcomes. Fundamental questions exist; who should judge, how could excessive rigidity in assessment and interference in clinical freedom be avoided? Those aspects of performance which are easily measured are not necessarily those of most importance to health care. Indeed consumer surveys show that the elements of care most significant to doctors are not always the same as those which matter to their patients. Should the same standards apply in the inner cities as in rural areas? Is there a problem of confidentiality? If money is to be used as well as the professional incentives of pride in one's work, an incentive needs to be devised not only to reward the good, but also to encourage all doctors to provide better standards of care. There are lessons to be learned from industry where rewards are seldom restricted to an elite, so that they are not seen as out of reach and irrelevant to the large majority of the staff on whose performance the well being of the organisation depends.

Such issues must be explored. But because they reach the heart of professional practice, doctors should take a lead. The problem of quality assessment has not been solved but it is not insoluble. The issue is now on the public agenda; there was support from consumer organisations as well as the profession for the idea of performance related pay. Commentators have suggested that there is a need for an incentive to innovate, evaluate and improve patient care. The tide is in the right direction and the way ahead may be for the profession and the health departments to enter into constructive discussions. Practice of the highest quality is more widespread than it has ever been, with the rising quality of entrants, the impact of compulsory vocational training and academic departments of general practice, the introduction of clinics for women and children, increased use of information technology and improvement of premises. What is now necessary is to raise the standard of all practices to that of the best.

References

1 Butler J. List size, standards and performance in general practice: a pilot study. In: Pendleton D, Schofield T, Marinker M, eds. *In pursuit of quality: approaches to performance review in general practice*. London: Royal College of General Practitioners, 1986: 85–95.
2 Metcalfe D. Variations in process in primary care. In: Pendleton D, Schofield T, Marinker M, eds. *In pursuit of quality: approaches to performance review in general practice*. London: Royal College of General Practitioners, 1986: 96–112.
3 Department of Health and Social Security, Welsh Office, Northern Ireland Office, Scottish Office. *Primary health care: an agenda for discussion*. London: HMSO, 1986. (Cmnd 9771).
4 Department of Health and Society Security. *Neighbourhood nursing: a focus for care: report of the Community Nursing Review*. London: HMSO, 1986. Chairman: Mrs J Cumberlege.

6.   CLINICAL SERVICES

(a) Committee on Safety of Medicines

(i) Terms of reference

The Committee on Safety of Medicines (CSM) was established in 1970 under Section 4 of the Medicines Act 1968. Its terms of reference are:

> To give advice with respect to safety, quality and and efficacy in relation to human use of any substances or article (not being an instrument, apparatus or appliance) to which any provision of the Medicines Act 1968 is applicable.

> To promote the collection and investigation of information relating to adverse reactions or the purpose of enabling such advice to be given.

(ii) Meetings

The Committee held 11 meetings during 1986. Two 2-day meetings, in May and September, were necessary to enable the Committee to complete its business.

(iii) Consideration of applications

Table 6.1 provides a statistical summary of applications for product licences (PLs) and clinical trial certificates (CTs) considered by the Committee during 1986.

Table 6.1: *CSM — 1986 Applications**

	Product Licences		Clinical Trial Certificates	
First Consideration by CSM				
Grant advised	30	(32)	9	(6)
Grant provisionally not advised	47	(87)	1	(2)
Advice following hearings and written representations				
Hearings — Grant advised	7	(5)	3	(1)
Hearings — Grant not advised	5	(5)	0	(0)
Written representations — Grant advised	17	(16)	0	(0)
Written representations — Grant not advised	3	(13)	1	(0)

*1985 figures are given in brackets.

The total number of applications referred to the Committee for its advice in 1986 was about one-third fewer than in recent years. The reason for this may have partly been a reflection of a temporary manpower shortage in the medical secretariat to the Committee, which resulted in very few applications being assessed for presentation to the Committee in the last few months of 1986. Of the product licence applications which were considered by the Committee for the first time in 1986 39% were considered to be satisfactory for the grant of a licence, which compares with an average of 28% over the 3 preceeding years.

(iv) Advice to Licensing Authority

In addition to applications for new products, the Committee gave advice to the Licensing Authority about a number of marketed products during 1986, including:

(a)   *Reye's syndrome and aspirin* — The Committee was concerned about a possible link between aspirin ingestion in children and Reye's Syndrome. The Chairman wrote to all doctors, dentists and pharmacists on 10 June 1986 advising that aspirin should not be given to children under 12 years of age unless specifically indicated. Further information was published in the *'CSM Update'* series in the *British Medical Journal*. Companies voluntarily removed from sale all paediatric aspirin-containing products, and the Aspirin Foundation conducted a publicity campaign aimed at parents.

(b)   *Halothane* — the Committee obtained the co-operation of manufacturers in strengthening the warnings of hepatic toxicity associated with the use of this anaesthetic, and lengthening the recommended interval between exposures to it. The Committee's concern was explained in *Current Problems No 18* (September 1986).

(c)   *Desensitising vaccines* — The Chairman wrote to all doctors on 8 October 1986 to warn them that because of the possibility of anaphylaxis following administration of desensitising vaccines (allergen extracts), such treatment should be given only where full resuscitation facilities were available and that patients should be kept under medical observation for at least 2 hours. Further information was published in the *'CSM Update'* series. Licensing action continues into 1987.

(d)   *Danthron* — the Committee considered that licensing action might be necessary because of concern about the possible risk of mutagenicity and carcinogenicity following reports of animal experiments in Japan. Action is continuing into 1987.

(e)   *Other Licensing Action* — after careful consideration of all the evidence available, including its own adverse reactions reports, the Committee advised that variations should be made to the product particulars of a number of product licences in 1986. In most cases these variations were carried out with the agreement and co-operation of the companies concerned, obviating the need for official regulatory action. In some cases the companies wrote to doctors and pharmacists, with the knowledge of the Committee, informing them of the changes.

The Committee continued to keep under consideration a number of important issues including the safety of all blood-derived products from contamination with HIV virus, the safety of non-steroidal anti-inflammatory drugs, and published reports linking oral contraceptive use with hepato-cellular and breast cancer.

(v) Communications with doctors and pharmacists

Three editions of *Current Problems*, the Committee's drug safety information sheet for doctors and pharmacists, were issued in February, May and September

1986. Two *'Dear Doctor'* letters were sent, on Reye's syndrome and on desensitising vaccines (see above). The *'CSM Update'* monthly feature continued through the year.

(vi) Adverse reactions

Adverse reactions to medicinal products are reported to the CSM on a voluntary basis by doctors and dentists under the yellow card scheme. Reports are also received from pharmaceutical companies and other professional sources. The Committee very much appreciates the co-operation of those who submit reports.

In 1986 yellow slips were included in FP10 pads and in the British National Formulary, providing clinicians with an alternative source of reporting forms. They have proved popular and accounted for 28% of the reports received in the last 8 months of 1986.

Table 6.2 shows the number of reports received since 1980; 1986 saw the highest ever annual total of reports, an increase of 23% over 1985.

Table 6.2: *Reports of suspected adverse reactions received for registration*

1980	10,179
1981	13,032
1982	10,922
1983	12,689
1984	12,163
1985	12,652
1986	15,527

(vii) Adverse Reactions Working party

The Committee's Adverse Reactions Working Party published a second report, on post-marketing surveillance, on 31 January 1986. Details of the recommendations and the working party's membership were given in the 1985 Annual Report of the CSM.

(viii) Electronic reporting of adverse reactions

The Committee's pilot project into the use of view data equipment in reporting adverse reactions continued during the year. No decisions were taken on its future.

(ix) Adverse reactions reporting by pharmacists

The Committee agreed to meet the Pharmaceutical Society of Great Britain to discuss the possibility of a pilot trial of adverse reaction reporting by community pharmacists. The Committee also agreed to the development of protocol for the involvement of hospital pharmacists in increasing adverse reaction reporting, following on from the successful experience at the Royal Liverpool Hospital.

(b) Hospital services

(i) Supra regional clinical services

Since the Report for 1985 (page 76) 11 applications have been considered by the Advisory Group for Supra regional clinical services. After due consideration the Advisory Group concluded that 10 of the services did not meet the criteria and recommended that the applications be rejected. One application is still under consideration.

(ii) Heart transplantation

This Report for 1985 (page 76) drew attention to the designation of heart transplantation as a supra regional service. The designated units were at Papworth, Harefield and Newcastle. During 1986 the Advisory Group recommended that a limited number of cardiac transplant operations should be performed on children at Great Ormond Street as an extension of the Papworth programme. The Advisory Group also foresaw a gradual expansion of heart transplantation as resources allowed, and Health Authorities were invited to submit applications for units they wished to be considered as a fourth heart transplant centre. Applications have now been received and are under consideration. In the 5 year period up to 31 December 1986 the number of transplantations carried out were as follows: hearts 518, heart and lungs 99, and lungs 3.

(iii) Liver transplantations

The Advisory Group recommended that a further unit should be added to the units mentioned in *this Report* for 1985 (page 76). The Secretary of State accepted the recommendation that the additional unit should be at Leeds. The number of liver transplantations carried out in the 5 years up to the 31 December 1986 was 307.

(iv) Paediatric end stage renal failure

During 1986 the Advisory Group received a report of a working party of the Royal College of Physicians on paediatric end stage renal failure services. The working party recommended that an additional centre be established at Nottingham. The Advisory Group recommended to the Secretary of State that the treatment of end stage renal failure in children would in the longer term best be provided on a regional rather than on a supra regional basis. The Secretary of State agreed in principle that 1987–88 should be the last year during which the service would be designated under the supra regional services arrangements.

(v) Lithotripsy

A major advance has been achieved in the last few years in the treatment of many patients who have kidney stones. The Lithotripter provides a non-invasive method for dispersing stones by subjecting them to focussed shock waves. This method may either be used alone or in conjunction with other techniques and results in considerable benefit for patients in that major surgery is not required.

A first generation lithotripter was installed in St Thomas's Hospital in March 1985 in conjunction with BUPA. Considerable experience in the provision of this form of treatment in the NHS has been achieved. This knowledge, taken in conjunction with the introduction of second generation machines, led to a Ministerial announcement that the lithotripsy service should develop on a Regional basis.

(c) The renewal of certificates granted under the Medicines (Administration of Radioactive Substances) Regulations (1978)

A doctor or a dentist who wishes to be able to adminster a radioactive medicinal product to a person requires a certificate issued by Ministers. Ministers are advised by the Administration of Radioactive Substances Advisory Committee. For diagnostic and therapeutic purposes certificates are issued for 5 years; for research purposes for up to 2 years.

The first certificates under the Medicines (Administration of Radioactive Substances) Regulations 1978 were issued to doctors and dentists in 1980 — 858 certificates were issued in 1980, 298 in 1981, 336 in 1982, 299 in 1983, 304 in 1984, 272, in 1985, 373 in 1986 and 102 to date in 1987. 1985 saw the need to re-certificate many of those who had been originally granted certificates in 1980 as well as the need to continue issuing new certificates. It was decided to automate as much of the certification procedure as possible. The software was written in-house using a relational database. While it has not been possible to automate as much of the certification procedure as had been hoped, it has been possible to conduct the exercise involving the renewal of certificates concurrently with the issue of new certificates without any increase in the number of staff providing the Secretariat for the Administration of Radioactive Substances Advisory Committee.

(d) EC Directive on protection of patients from medical uses of radiation

In September 1984 the Council of the European Communities adopted EC Directive 84/466/Euratom which lays down basic measures for the radiation protection of people undergoing medical examination or treatment. The purpose of the Directive is to protect people against over-exposure to, or unskilled application of, diagnostic X-rays, radiotherapy and radioactive medicinal products. The Directive is binding on all Member States of the European Community and legislation is required to implement it. It is proposed to supplement existing legislation, and give legislative backing to existing good practice, by making Regulations under the European Communities Act 1972.

The main requirements of the Directive are that:

(1)   The various types of activity leading to exposures to radiation should be medically justified, and that individual exposures should be as low as reasonably achievable;

(2)   Such exposures should be carried out by qualified practitioners who have received training and achieved competence in both the radiological techniques they practice and in radiation protection;

(3)   There should be adequate quality control of the equipment used; and

(4)   The services of a medical physicist should be available to radiotherapy and nuclear medicine departments.

The NHS and the professions were formally consulted about the draft Regulations in June 1986. Following consultation the draft Regulations have been revised. It is proposed that the Ionising Radiations (Protection of Persons Undergoing Medical Examination or Treatment) Regulations will come into force in 1987.

(e) Breast cancer screening

Following the publication of the Swedish prospective study[1] of the clinical value of breast cancer screening in April 1985, the then Minister for Health, on behalf of the UK Health Ministers, set up a Working Group chaired by Professor Sir Patrick Forrest to consider UK policy on breast cancer screening.

The Working Group took evidence from 40 invited experts and in its Interim Report concluded from the principal overseas trials that deaths from breast cancer in women aged 50–64 years who are offered screening by mammography could be reduced by one-third or more.

The Group's Final Report (November 1986) was considered by Ministers and on the 25 February 1987 the Secretary of State announced the Government's acceptance of the proposals made in the Report and the decision to introduce a national breast cancer screening service. The essential features are screening every 3 years for women in the age-group 50–64 years. Women over the age of 64 years will be offered screening on demand. Women under the age of 50 years will require a GP referral letter either to a consultant surgeon or for direct-access mammography.

By March 1988 each Region is expected to have established one screening centre and one team for the assessment and management of screen-detected abnormalities. Four of these initial 14 centres will be national training centres — at Guildford, at Nottingham, at South Manchester and at King's College Hospital, London. Funds have been made available to cover the cost of setting up and operating call and recall, the basic screening centre, assessment, diagnosis and such additional treatment as will be required during the initial screening period. Additional allocations have been made to cover the cost of the 4 training centres providing the national training facility. As well as facilities for training radiologists and radiographers, the national training centres will be expected to provide for the training of other health professionals.

The Forrest report divides the screening procedure into 4 stages:

(1)   The basic screen to detect an abnormality, which may or may not be cancer;

(2)   The assessment of abnormality to detect whether a surgical biopsy is required;

(3)   Definitive diagnosis by biopsy and the laboratory examintion of the removed tissue; and

(4)   Treatment of screen-detected cancers.

Basic screening method

The Report concludes that high quality single medio-lateral oblique view mammography is the preferred basic screening method for mass population screening. The Working Group also concluded that there is no evidence that clinical examination or breast self-examination is effective when used alone. These methods may have some value when used in combination with mammography but their contribution requires further assessment. The Report, nevertheless, does recognise the contribution of breast self-examination to earlier diagnosis and states that lack of evidence on its effectiveness should not discourage women from practising breast examination.

Assessment

The Report states that the specialised techniques required for the assessment of screen-detected abnormalities are best carried out by a skilled multidisciplinary team, either within a hospital or in a clinic in the community. A team should consist of a clinician, a radiologist and a pathologist all trained in the diagnosis of breast disease. They should be supported by a radiographer and a nurse, both trained in the specialist skills required to care for women who may have cancer, and a receptionist.

Diagnosis and treatment

The Report recommends that biopsies of impalpable screen-detected abnormalities should, wherever possible, be performed by a specialist breast team experienced in the surgical, radiological and pathological skills necessary for their localisation. Specialist breast teams should be experienced in the various treatment options for small cancers. They are also more likely to be aware of women's anxieties about breast biopsy and to have nurses specially trained to inform and support the women.

It is recognised that screening will increase the demand for biopsy and treatment. This will be greatest during the initial screen. The Report estimates that during this period the extra number of biopsies that will be generated by each basic screening centre, that is for each half million population, will be between 2 and 3 a week. Once the initial screen is completed the number should fall to one extra per week. As far as treatment is concerned, it is estimated that there would be less than one extra case each week during the initial period after which numbers should fall back towards the normally expected incidence.

Reference

[1] Tabar L, Fagerberg C J G, Gad A, Baldetorp L et al. Reduction in mortality from breast cancer after mass screening with mammography. Randomised trial from the Breast Cancer Screening Group of the Swedish National Board of Health and Welfare, *Lancet* 1985; 1: 829–32.

(f) Cervical cancer screening

Several organisations issued reports on this subject during the year[1-4]. The evaluation of screening programmes in 8 countries from the International Agency for Research on Cancer was of particular importance. The study estimated the risks of cervical cancer associated with different screening policies. The reduction of cancer of the cervix in women screened every 5 years between the ages of 35 and 64 years was found to be 70%; while screening at this interval between the ages of 20 and 64 years resulted in a reduction of 84%. Changing from 5-yearly to 3-yearly screening could result in a further reduction of 7% but would involve a large increase in laboratory workload.

These figures confirm the importance of the priority already being given in the UK to increasing the uptake of screening substantially. It is regrettable that the current position in this country remains that most women presenting with cancer of the cervix have never had a smear test. Health Authorities have been asked to ensure that computerised call and recall schemes to trigger the sending of personal screening invitations to women are implemented no later than 31 March 1988. They have also been asked to take steps to improve laboratory services so as to eliminate backlogs of unexamined smears.

References

[1] IARC working group on evaluation of cervical cancer screening programmes. *Screening for squamous cervical cancer: Duration of law risk after negative results of cervical cytology and its implication for screening policies. Br Med J* 1986; **293:** 659–64.

[2] World Health Organisation. Control of cancer of the cervix uteri. *Bull WHO* 1986; **64:** 607–18.

[3] *Cervical cancer and screening in Great Britain: report of the British Medical Association.* British Medical Association. Board of Science and Education. London, 1986.

[4] ICRF Coordinating Committee on Cervical Screening. The management of a cervical screening programme: a statement (October 1985). *Community Med* 1986; **8:** 179–84.

(g) 'Helping people with special needs in the community'

"Community Care is a matter of marshalling resources, sharing responsibilities, and combining skills to achieve good quality modern services to meet the actual needs of real people, in ways those people find acceptable and in places which encourage rather than prevent normal living".

Thus did the Government in its response[1] to the Report of the Social Services Committee on Community Care with Special Reference to Adult Mentally Ill and Mentally Handicapped People endorse community care as a philosophy. A timely reminder was also given that 'community care is not something new. It has been preached and practiced for a long time' and many people with many different problems, not only in the field of mental health, have for a long time been cared for outside of institutions and in many different ways.

Care in the community is not a cheap alternative to institutional care, nor is it a simple option to implement. Seductive assumptions that simply being outside rather than in an institution will automatically lead to less disability and a better quality of life cannot be sustained. To meet the actual needs of real people requires the development of a range of provision comprehensively planned and developed to meet a broad spectrum of individual needs. 'No single authority could embrace all this'[2] and services have to be planned jointly by health and local authorities, and involve voluntary organisations.

The bounds of what is possible are still being explored for some of the most severely disabled groups, and new patterns of service utilising new professional skills delivered in new contexts are being developed. When the extent of the potential is so uncertain it is essential that flexibility is built into developing services and that these are continuously monitored. There are particular challenges for managers in understanding the variety of needs, and in facilitating and supporting the complex multi-disciplinary networks which are required to meet the identified needs. In the management of mentally handicapped people some health authorities have developed and implemented policies on risk taking. Ensuring the safety and security of individuals, of other clients, or patients, of carers and of the general public has to be weighed against individual needs. As we grow up, taking part in everyday life and learning from our mistakes is, for all of us, an important part of learning to cope with life. Risk taking is a necessary element of this process. Mentally handicapped people also need to learn in this way but in the past the care offered in institutional settings has often been over-protective, and over concerned, with avoiding difficult life situations rather than helping people to learn without embarrassment or distress to others, without putting themselves or others at risk of physical harm, and without damage to property. Individual treatment plans for mentally handicapped people should therefore have regard to the need to take carefully considered risks with safeguards where appropriate, and there this is clearly seen to be in the interests of the development and well being of the individual.

As experience is gained from the planning, developing and running of services in the community so particular issues have become highlighted — some very specific to particular groups, others common to many groups. There is need to identify and provide networks of services for people who are disabled by long-term mental illness, for the frail elderly, and for people who are sensorally handicapped.

Attention has to be given to understanding and responding to people with very special needs. To mentally handicapped people with behaviour disorders or a mental illness, to brain damaged young adults, to disturbed adolescents, to multi-handicapped people (including those who are deaf and dumb) and to people who suffer from incontinence. Thought also needs to be given to those who may have difficulty gaining access to, and communicating with services, such as people who are homeless, or members of ethnic minorities.

Account must be taken of the burden of care, arising from a wide range of disabilities, which is placed on families and other carers.

(i) The care of chronically mentally ill people

Despite advances in methods of treatment and the provision of better, more local services, it sadly remains a fact that mental illness often leads to long-term disability. Johnstone *et al*[3] have shown that less than 20% of patients suffering from schizophrenia discharged from hospital were symptom free at follow-up. The increasing number of very elderly people in the population means that we will be faced with a much greater number of people needing care for the problems of dementia.

The need to plan services in the light of the special needs of those people who are chronically disabled by mental illness was recognised in *Better Services for the Mentally Ill*[4] and the importance of this group was clearly emphasised in the Government's Response to the Social Services Committee Report on Community Care[1]. The Government accepted the Committee's view that "the real test of services is not whether they provide adequately for those who least need them, but whether they provide well for those who most need them"[2]. Those who are chronically disabled by mental illness are a major group in the category of "most needing help".

The Government Response also recognised "the need to avoid developing services for those with mild disorders at the expense of those with more serious disorders". And that such "shift of balance is always a risk as more professional work is done in the community where milder forms of disorder are more prevalent . . .".

In the past much of the care for those people who are chronically disabled by mental illness has been provided in traditional multi-district mental illness hospitals. For many years however an increasing proportion of patients have been considered to be better treated out of hospital and this trend was greatly accelerated by the advent of the major psycholeptic drugs in the 1950s, providing relief of symptoms which were previously severely disabling. Research has suggested[5] that there are now getting on for 100,000 people severely disabled by mental illness in the community. In 1985 there where also nearly 64,000 patients resident in mental illness hospitals and units. Of these over 36,000 had been in hospital for more than 1 year. Study of regional strategic plans suggests that a further 5,000 severely disabled patients are likely to be discharged over the 10 year strategic planning period.

Present policy calls for a comprehensive service for mental illness in each health district. The elements of a comprehensive district service especially relevant to those chronically disabled by mental illness are likely to include residential, occupational, and treatment elements. Although some patients will need longer term hospital care or will be best suited by new styles of care such as a hospital hostel[5,6] many others, if given the information with which to make reasoned choices will prefer to live in smaller groups or in their own homes[7]. It is probable that even of those more severely disabled the majority live in their own homes or with their families. The need for a wide range of types of accommodation has been suggested[8].

Facilities offering daytime occupation for chronically disabled people are of importance in helping the individual to structure the day, to meet others, and to preserve or regain work skills. Treatment may involve physical treatments, but will certainly call for the skilled use of supportive techniques to help the person cope with the problems of disabilities. Community psychiatric nurses and also clinical psychologists both have important roles to play here. Services for those people who are chronically disabled and living in the community are also important and special consideration needs to be given to problems of co-ordination across agencies, health, social services, local authority housing, housing associations, and voluntary bodies. Services should particularly endeavour to ensure continuity of care and that the care given varies appropriately as the person needs change. The computer based psychiatric service registers that some districts are developing are examples of attempts to meet these needs; some of these are projects supported by the Department's 'Helping the Community to Care' Initiative and reports on them will be available by the end of 1987. The necessity of ensuring appropriateness and continuity is also being addressed by experiments in the use of care managers[9].

Among those people who are chronically disabled by mental illness are some groups which need special consideration. A high incidence of mental illness is reported among those living rough and in hostels for the homeless, and conventional service delivery often does not appear adequately to meet the needs of this group. Experiments in psychiatric health care delivery to this group may show a way forward.

Concern has also been expressed that a proportion of those with chronic mental illness and disability tend to find their way in and out of prison. A working group has been set up to look at the needs of these patients and to look at ways to ensure that they get placed in mental health care, where appropriate, rather than in prison; that, while in prison, their needs can be met: and perhaps most importantly that prior to discharge from prison, ways can be sought to link those needing continuing treatment and support with local mental health services.

(ii) The needs of brain damaged young adults

In its Report *'Physical Disabilities in 1986 and Beyond'* published in July 1986, the Royal College of Physicians gave attention to the disabilities arising from head injury[10]. During both the acute and recovery phases people with head injury tend to be dispersed among many different hospital wards and departments, as well as community services. Many will be at home with their families and may not be identified as suffering from the consequences of head injury or necessarily be in contact with appropriate services. It is therefore difficult to obtain good information on the overall prevalence, characteristics, and natural history of these disabilities. Nevertheless it has been estimated that there will

101

be approximately 34 major head injuries occurring each year in an average health district, and that about 8 of these will be left with severe permanent disability. Less than 40% of these problems result from road traffic accidents and a substantial proportion are due to a variety of causes, such as assaults, toxic effects, anorexia, and infections. Preventive action, although important, is thus not simply a matter of reducing the risks arising from road traffic accidents. The MRC Co-ordinating Group on the Rehabilitation of The Acutely Brain Damaged Adult[11] estimated the prevalence of severe head injury disability at about 150 per 100,000 population. This number may not be great but being a youthful population — around 50% are under the age of 20 years — it can be expected that they will survive for many years. The brain lesions are typically widespread and therefore the resulting disabilities tend to be multiple and often include emotional, cognitive, and behavioural impairments, so that although there are frequently potentials for rehabilitation, for the development of skills, and for the modification of anti-social or violent behaviour the management of each individual case can be complex.

The Report of the Royal College of Physicians drew attention to a lack of awareness by health authorities of the needs of this comparatively small group and to the difficulties of developing expertise among staff when so many individuals present sporadically to different services. Few health districts have developed facilities for their management.

Of concern also is the fact that long-term disabilities are not limited to those recovering from severe head injury, but are also encountered among the much larger groups of people recovering from moderate to mild injury[12]. High levels of cognitive, emotional, and behavioural disorders have been reported[13] among survivors and these problems show little tendency to spontaneous improvement over time. These difficulties are not always understood or easily tolerated by rehabilitative services, and problems arise because inattentiveness and loss of emotional control may be misinterpreted as deliberate obstruction or poor motivation unless there is sufficient experience and level of awareness among staff, or unless there is access to support from staff of other services who have these skills. Relatives find the psychiatric symptoms a particularly stressful burden to accept[13] but may not always be in contact with or helped by support services[14].

A wide range of disciplines and services can be identified as having potential roles to play — for example neurology and neurosurgery, psychiatry, clinical psychology, rehabilitative medicine, orthopaedics, services for the elderly, occupational therapy, speech therapy, physiotherapy, community nursing, and community psychiatric nursing. The MRC Group pointed to the importance of early assessment, on-going assessment, and long-term care arrangements. These clearly require team work and good co-ordination between services, but as the Royal College of Physicians points out there is insufficient evidence as yet to identify the features of a model service. Nevertheless many of the services within a health district but particularly psychiatry, neurosurgery, and rehabilitation, need to be aware of the problems posed by these individuals and to contribute to the rehabilitation and support provided by them.

The Royal College of Physicians Report makes a number of recommendations among which are that every health authority should have a written policy for the management of head injury, that statistics should be kept, and that there should be a named consultant in each health district who would be in charge of head injury recovery services. It suggests that patients in the early recovery phase should be managed on wards where staff are fully trained, but that this might necessitate mixing them with patients who have allied neurological disabilities such as stroke or multiple sclerosis.

The Report draws attention to the importance of follow-up and also of day care. With respect to day care the point is made that it is not suitable for younger patients to be managed in a geriatric day hospital. This statement highlights a dilemma because although brain damaged young adults may have some disabilities in common with, for example, people who are elderly and disabled, people who are chronically mentally ill, or people who are mentally handicapped they also have other features which distinguish them, and this may necessitate other forms of care and other therapeutic interventions. Being placed with other client groups can be a source of distress for individuals and for their families. On the other hand the numbers may be insufficient to justify a special facility for this group at a district level while provision at a regional or sub-regional level may be so remote that links with local services are more difficult to develop or maintain.

Co-ordination of service, early and on-going multi-disciplinary assessment, the development of professional skills and the facilitation of access to these may be of equal or even greater importance than the development of special units. It is for consideration whether mental health services which should also be thinking in terms of a named consultant and a numbed clinical psychologist to liaise with other district services in the development of a more appropriate response to brain damaged young adults.

Support for families and for brain damaged people is also advocated by Headway, a voluntary organisation grant aided by the Department. In March 1987 Headway ran a one day conference to consider the implications for service providers of the recommendation of health injury services contained in the Royal College of Physicians Report. Also anticipated during 1987 is a Report from the Medical Disability Society on this subject which will helpfully include more detailed information on incidence and prevalence as a basis for further discussion of the needs of brain damaged young adults.

(iii) The needs of disturbed adolescents

The publication of the Health Advisory Service *'Bridges Over Troubled Water'*[15], on services for disturbed adolescents, reinforces the need for a wide network of statutory and voluntary services to be involved in the co-ordinated planning and provision of flexible local services for this group.

Adolescence is often a disturbed and disturbing time. The Report stated that "more than for any other group an appropriate response cannot be the province in isolation of any one agency" and provided 11 principles on which a good service should be based, which include the need for separate consideration and provision for this age-group (13–18 years), a clear understanding and awareness of the ethical legal issues involved in working with adolescents and their families, and the need for accessible and acceptable services and sustained support.

Support for families is of vital importance. The Report indicates how difficult it may be for both young people and their families to identify where to turn for help, and how sometimes the help offered seems to ignore the main problem. The general practitioner has a key role, both in providing an important first contact, and as a source of continued support, particularly for the parents.

Within the wide spectrum of need, groups which are frequently not receiving proper attention are older adolescents, and those with mental handicap, with associated physical and sensory handicap, and with autism.

The Report is commended as a useful basis on which to develop services for this vulnerable group.

(iv) The problems of people who are both deaf and blind

The needs of people with a combination of different impairments, whether physical, sensory or mental, raise special difficulties for service providers. A flexible approach and close collaboration between the various professions providing care and treatment are of vital importance if a multi-handicapped person is to reach optimum levels of achievement.

People who are both deaf and blind form a group with very specialised needs. The precise number of deaf-blind people in England is not known but estimates suggest that there may be about 1,200 children under 16 years old, 2,500 young adults — including the 'bulge' of rubella handicapped people from the epidemic in the early 1960's — and 5,000 elderly people.

Services need to be individually tailored depending on age, needs and abilities. The needs of congenitally handicapped people are not necessarily the same as those of adventitiously deaf-blind people. A fundamental task is the development of communication skills. Other forms of assistance, such as training in the use of residual hearing or sight, the development of physical co-ordination and other senses, mobility and orientation training, and the provision of a guide/helper/interpreter, are also important.

Statutory service providers have so far found it difficult to help deaf-blind people, perhaps partly, and as with other special needs groups because relatively few will reside within the bounds of any one health or local authority. Voluntary organisations — in particular SENSE (the national Deaf-Blind and Rubella Association) and the National Deaf Blind Helpers League — have played an increasingly important role, not only in heightening awareness of deaf-blindness and conditions such as Usher's Syndrome (in which congenitally deaf people progressively lose their sight) but also in providing some services; residential and rehabilitation facilites; counselling and support for families and for the professions working with deaf-blind people. For practical reasons the proportion of deaf-blind people who can be helped directly by voluntary organisations is limited. However, statutory service providers can draw upon the expertise acquired by the voluntary organisations to try to ensure that the needs for service of people who are deaf-blind and of their families are properly assessed and met, either by adapting existing facilities or by arranging specialised help.

(v) The needs of mentally handicapped people with problem behaviours or mental illness

The shift in the balance of care for mentally handicapped people away from hospital provision towards non-institutional care is gathering pace, and as it does so the importance of carefully assessing the needs of individuals and planning for future provision to meet those needs has become clearer.

Some mentally handicapped people have very special needs and many of these were addressed in the Report of a DHSS Study Team 'Helping Mentally Handicapped People with Special Problems' which was issued in 1984[16]. This demonstrated the very wide spectrum of special needs and looked in detail at many of them. One area of special need — that posed by mental illness and behavioural disturbances — was largely seen as beyond the scope of the team. With the passage of time it is clear that these problems pose particular difficulties for those who are now planning and developing services for mentally handicapped people.

Problem behaviours, abnormal reactions, and mental illness do occur in some mentally handicapped people and have many causes ranging from physical damage to the central nervous system, through the effects of the particular circumstances and vulnerabilities of mentally handicapped people, to causes of similar problems occurring in the rest of the population. Whatever the cause these problems present particular challenges to a range of services and require careful and sensitive planning to meet individual needs if they are to be successfully prevented or treated.

During the latter half of 1986 a Departmental Team commenced a Study which involves both visits to look at the range of services which try to meet these needs, and a series of workshops with practitioners in the field to discuss and refine some of the issues involved.

Although each mentally handicapped person has very specific needs which should be addressed individually it has proved helpful to planners to have regard to the needs arising from clusters of similar types of problem: mentally handicapped people who are also mentally ill; profoundly and severely mentally handicapped people with behaviour disorders, including autistic behaviours; mildly mentally handicapped people who present with delinquent behaviour, including autistic behaviours and who may be offenders; mildly to moderately handicapped people who for much of the time cope well but who present with episodes of problem behaviours.

It seems likely that as comprehensive and effective networks of services become established, and given time, all but the most severe of these problems may be satisfactorily managed, treated, and in many cases ameliorated within the range of settings in the community where mentally handicapped people with these problems can be expected to live. To meet the needs of these people services will require adequate numbers of staff with appropriate skills, backed up by support networks which can offer special expertise in the prevention, assessment, and treatment, of them. The range of expertise will include the skills, among others, of clinical psychologists, mental handicap nurses, social workers, speech therapists, and psychiatrists.

In the meantime and as these services develop over the next few years, it is anticipated that existing mental handicap hospitals and units will have to treat and care for a higher proportion of these problems among their residents. Even in the longer term and when a comprehensive and more effective range of services which do have access to appropriate skills has been developed there is every reason to expect that there will remain a relatively small number of people with severe problems for whom specialist medical and nursing treatment will have to be provided in specialised residential health care settings. The exact number of mentally handicapped people requiring this special level of care is not known, it could well become smaller as services develop and become more effective and as intervention skills improve. The number of individuals in some of the groups identified may be so small that services for them may need to be planned at a supra-district, or even regional level. This will necessitate giving particular attention to the problem of liaison and co-ordination with local services.

It seems likely that the manpower requirements for the most difficult problems will be on the high side but the pattern of special service provision which develops will vary according to particular local needs and circumstances.

No matter what pattern of services emerges it must be seen as part of an overall network of services which is flexible and which tries to respond to individual needs. It must develop good links with community services, with primary care services, with educational services, and with mental illness services, and be able to work flexibly with them. It will require adequate staffing levels and a range of professional skills.

The Department's Team will continue the Study in 1987 and intends to highlight the issues, and consider further the range of appropriate responses to meet these challenging problems.

(vi) Meeting the needs of ethnic minorities in the community

Authorities with large ethnic minority populations are in general aware of the dietary, social, family, and other issues which can arise for them and may call on their own ethnic minority staff for special insight and help with language difficulties. They may thus be well placed to give some help to authorities with less experience. Approved social worker training usually deals with this subject. Transcultural psychiatry is being developed in various places; and the Department is giving support to one London based service. The mental health needs of black children and young black adults merit particular attention.

All professional staff whose daily work brings them into contact with members of ethnic minorities need training in this area if they are to provide a relevant service. Local authorities often provide or have access to interpreters; their training needs are particularly important when dealing with such problems as suspected mental illness. A recent National Social Service Inspection of 8 local authorities threw up one example of an unqualified social worker from an ethnic minority who was funded by Section 11 monies, and appointed to support hospital social work colleagues in looking at the special mental health needs of ethnic minority groups.

(vii) Hypothermia and excess winter mortality in the elderly

The spell of very cold weather early on in the year led, predictably, to a marked increase in the number of registrations of deaths of people over 65 which were associated with hypothermia. Overall the number of such deaths during the whole of 1986 was little different from that during the previous year — 701 in England and Wales in 1986 compared with 709 in 1985.

The number of deaths recorded as associated with hypothermia is influenced not only by the actual incidence of the condition and associated fatalities, but it also reflects changes in awareness, improved diagnosis, certification practice and other factors. A much more meaningful indicator of the effects of cold weather on the elderly is the extent to which the overall mortality in the winter exceeds that in the summer — due, in the main, to an increased mortality from heart disease, strokes and chest infections. This so called 'excess winter mortality' is about 37,000 each year (in terms of a comparison between mortality in the winter and summer quarters); however it has decreased considerably in recent years, from about 69,000 in the early 1950s. The reasons for the decline are not fully understood.

In December 1986 the Government introduced improved arrangements for 'exceptionally cold weather payments' under the Supplementary Benefit System; these now provide for payments to be related to local temperatures.

(viii) The challenge of incontinence

The prevalence of adult incontinence of all degrees of severity in the population of the UK is estimated to be of the order of 2½ million. It can cause great personal and social difficulties and the costs both for individuals and for the statutory services are considerable. It is a particular burden for elderly sufferers and places heavy strains on their families. It can also be a precipitating factor in the admission of elderly people to residential or hospital care. Awareness of the important contribution which can be made by the correct management of incontinence and by the provision of appropriate, largely non-institutional, services has continued to grow. The number of continence advisers appointed by health authorities has also increased and this, together with the use of multi-disciplinary assessment procedures have had a beneficial effect. Recent Department initiatives have included an evaluation study of pads and garments, a critical review of research, a seminar for health and social service managers, and 2 projects to develop training and information materials for general practitioners, community nurses, social services staff, informal carers and people who suffer from incontinence.

(ix) The burden of families and other carers

The large majority of people in the priority care groups — that is people who are mentally ill, mentally handicapped, elderly, or physically disabled — live at home. Many will have special needs and some of these have been discussed above. We do not have firm figures on the total numbers who are dependent on the informal care provided by family members or other carers, but there seems little doubt that there are many thousands of families who accept often very heavy responsibilities and burdens in order to care for a family member in need. Within the domiciliary setting, therefore, help should be provided not only for the individual but also for the family and other informal carers.

There will be some for whom care by the family will not necessarily be the most appropriate response and, in assessing need, regard should be given not only to the quality of life of the individual but also to the quality of life of family and other carers. Section 8 of the Disabled Persons (Services, Consultation and Representation) Act 1986[17] requires that a local authority, in assessing the needs of a disabled person, should have regard for the ability of a carer, if there is one, to continue to provide such care on a regular basis.

There is some evidence[18] that the ability of carers to cope depends not only on the severity of the disability, but also the quality of the emotional relationships which have existed between the individual and his carers, and the extent to which emotional distress is part of the individual's reaction to his disabilities.

A series of newspaper articles on schizophrenia in 1984[19] graphically portrayed the burden which some forms of chronic mental illness can impose on carers as well as the levels of support which they require. These difficulties are recognised by the Department and in 1986 the Secretary of State announced that £6 million would be available over the next 3 years for development projects to establish or improve multi-disciplinary community orientated services for people with mental illness and their families. Each region was asked to submit one or more district based projects and by December 1986 central financial support had been approved for projects in 12 of the 14 health regions. The National Schizophrenia Fellowship, in its evidence to the House of Commons Select Committee on Community Care[2], put better information at the very top of the needs which carers have. Carers of other special needs groups also see information as important. The Department's *Helping the Community to Care* programme has funded the King's Fund to develop information packages for carers as well as those for whom they care.

Other factors influencing the quality of life and the burden on carers are the length of time the burden has to be carried, the continuous involvement and alertness needed by carers, and the repetitive nature of many of the tasks[18]. A good quality of life for carers cannot be inferred simply because they appear to be coping well and it is perhaps helpful to draw parallels with the 'burn-out' which has been described in the staff of those small isolated unsupported community projects who may be under considerable levels of stress over long periods of time.

We know that relatives often want to care for disabled members of their families and that they can be helped to make a therapeutic contribution[20]. The policy, occasionally followed in the past, of offering domiciliary help only to those people without family carers was poor practice and poor economics.

The parents of mentally handicapped people, for example, often have difficulty in 'letting-go' and accepting help. There is much to support the view that families are better able to cope when they have access to information and resources, appropriate professional and other supports, and access to respite care. One of the *Helping the Community to Care* projects is helping to develop, in 3 different areas, voluntary services which provide support for carers.

Services which include flexible arrangements for respite care will help families who want to care for a disabled relative to cope longer, and with more difficult problems than would otherwise be the case. This can take the form of regular arrangements, or be available on an *ad hoc* basis to cover special events, holidays, and family emergencies. It can take the form of residential or hospital care, 'drop-in' day care, more intensive domiciliary care or, as for some mentally handicapped children, can be provided through fostering schemes. For the frail elderly and the elderly mentally ill 'granny-sitting' schemes can afford important relief.

Access to these services may be less easy for some groups, such as ethnic minorities, while the respite facilities may not be able to tolerate some clients, for example, mentally handicapped people or elderly people who are behaviourly disturbed. Those planning services should not expect to be able to manage everyone in this way and should acknowledge the limits of carers, both initially and over time, as well as understanding that with appropriate support, thresholds can actually be raised.

The planning of services and support for carers in the community should involve health authorities, local authorities and voluntary organisations. The use of key workers, and the careful co-ordination of domiciliary services backed up by professional support, as in some community support schemes for the elderly, can do much to ensure that the most appropriate care is made available to individuals without confusion and overlap between different agencies and services. Intensive packets of domiciliary inputs, although seemingly costly may prove less expensive than other alternatives such as hospital care.

Carers should be involved in the planning of the particular packages of services for the individuals for whom they are caring. It is also for consideration whether they should be involved in some way in the planning of services overall particularly for those groups where caring is likely to be a major contribution over a long period of time. The National Council for Carers and Their Elderly Dependents, and the Association of Carers, both of whom are grant aided by the Department, are able to offer useful advice and experience in this field both to other carers and to those providing services.

The needs of elderly people for residental care

When independent living, or care by the family begin to look a less appropriate response to the care of an elderly person, a full assessment of need together with a realistic appraisal of alternative options should be part of any consideration for placement in residential care. During 1984 and 1985 the Department organised a series of seminars in different parts of the country which were attended by both NHS and Local Authority staff and which were aimed at encouraging a full multi-disciplinary assessment procedure for all elderly people referred for local authority residential care[21]. Special emphasis was placed on the importance of an adequate medical assessment of the health care needs of such elderly people. During 1986 this initiative was extended by the setting up of collaborative projects with 4 local authorities and their respective district health authorities.

Also during 1986 a Joint Central and Local Government Working Party was formed to look further at public financial support for people in local authority and private or voluntary residential homes. It will be making its Report to

Ministers and to the Local Authority Associations during 1987. At the same time the Department has put in hand similar work relating to the financial support of people in private or voluntary nursing homes.

References

1. The Department of Health and Social Security. Government response to the second report from the Social Services Committee. 1984–85 Session: community care: with special reference to adult mentally ill and mentally handicapped people. London: HMSO, 1985 (Cmnd 9674).

2. House of Commons. Social Services Committee. Community care with special reference to adult mentally ill and mentally handicapped people: second report from the Social Services Committee: session 1984–85. London: HMSO, 1985. Chairman Mrs Renee Short (HC13: Vols 1–III).

3. Johnstone E C, Owens D G C, Gold A, Crow T T, MacMillan J F. Schizophrenia patients discharged from hospital: A follow-up study. Br J Psychiatry 1984; 145: 586–90.

4. Department of Health and Social Security. Better services for the mentally ill. London: HMSO, 1975 (Cmnd 6233).

5. Sturt E, Wykes T, Creer C. Demographic social and clinical characteristics of the sample. In: Wing J K, ed. Long-term community care: experience in a London borough. Cambridge: Cambridge University Press, 1982. (Psychological medicine. Monograph Supplement 2.)

6. Goldberg D P, Bridges K, Cooper W, Hyde C, Sterling C, Wyatt R. Douglas House: A new type of hostel ward for chronic psychotic patients. 1985. Br J Psychiatry 1985; 147: 383–8.

7. Abrahamson D, Brenner D. Do long stay psychiatric patients want to leave hospital? Health Trends 1982; 14: 95–7.

8. Lovett A. A house for all reasons: The role of housing in community care. In Reed J, Lomas G, eds. Psychiatric services in the community. London: Croom Helm, 1984; 91–104.

9. Turner J C, Tenhoor W J. The NIMH community support program: Pilot to needed social reform. Schizophr Bull 1978; 4: 319–44.

10. Royal College of Physicians: Physical disability in 1986 and beyond: a report of the Royal College of Physicians. J Royal College Phys 1986; 20: 160–94.

11. Aitken C, Baddeley A, Bond M R, Brocklehurst J C, Brooks D N, Hewer R L, et al. Research aspects of rehabilitation after acute brain damage in adults. Lancet 1982; 2:1034–6.

12. Miller J D, Jones P A. The work of a regional head injury service. Lancet 1985; 1: 1141–4.

13. Mckinlay W W, Brooks D N, Bond M R. The short term outcome of severe blunt head injury as reported by relatives of the injured persons. J Neurol Neurosurg Psychiatry 1981; 44: 527–33.

14. Livingston M G. Assessment of need for co-ordinated approach in families with victims of head injury. Br Med J 1986; 293: 742–4.

15. Health Advisory Service. Bridges over troubled waters: a report from the NHS Health Advisory Service on services for disturbed adolescents. London: HMSO, 1986.

16. Department of Health and Social Security. Helping mentally handicapped people with special problems. Report of a DHSS Study Team. London: DHSS, 1984.

17. Disabled Persons (Services, Consultation and Representation) Act 1986.

18. Anderson R. The unremitting burden of carers. Br Med J 1987; 294: 73.

19. Wallace M. The tragedy of schizophrenia. The Times 1985 (16, 17, 18 Dec): 10 (col 1), 8 (col 1) 8 (col 1).

20. Kuipers L, Bebbington P. Relatives as a resource in the management of functional illness. Br J Psychiatry 1985; 147: 465–70.

21. Department of Health and Social Security. Assessment procedures for elderly people referred for local authority residential care: DHSS Social Services Inspectorate, 1985.

(h) Aspects of human reproduction

(i) Prenatal detection of fetal abnormalities

Over the past few years it has become possible to detect many more congenital abnormalities during pregnancy. Development of ultrasound scanning has made detailed study of fetal structure possible, and it is common practice for obstetricians to offer women an ultrasound scan at around 18 weeks of gestation. This may detect otherwise unsuspected structural abnormalities of the heart, kidneys, abdominal wall and skeleton. It may permit confirmation of the presence of abnormalities predicted by other means (eg neural tube defects strongly suspected because of high alpha-fetoprotein levels in the serum and amniotic fluid). As a result of these developments it is necessary to know the accuracy of ultrasound scanning in detecting fetal abnormalities. Research on this has begun. Antenatal detection of fetal abnormalities requires collaboration between several specialties. To achieve this the British Association of Paediatric Surgeons has set up a working group with representatives of the Royal College of Obstetricians and Gynaecologists, the Royal Collge of Pathologists, the Royal College of Radiologists and the British Paediatric Association which will be looking particularly at the clinical management of fetal abnormalities in relation to ultrasound scanning.

Until recently detection of chromosomal and genetic abnormalities by examining fetal cells has not been possible before 16 weeks of gestation. This has been because cells could only be obtained by amniocentesis. Therefore, if termination of pregnancy has then been offered and accepted, the special problems of mid-trimester abortion have had to be faced by the woman. However, the technique of chorionic villus sampling at 8 weeks of gestation now makes it possible to obtain cells of fetal origin which may be examined for chromosomal and genetic abnormalities at a much earlier stage. The sampling is done under ultrasound visualisation, so an important factor in its development has been the high resolution image which ultrasound can now achieve. During 1986 a trial of the safety and effectiveness of chorionic villus sampling began, funded by the MRC.

Despite the emergency of the techniques referred to above there are some fetal abnormalities which can only be detected by examining fetal blood, or by other special diagnostic methods. These are usually of relevance only when previous children are known to have been affected. Recognition of the need for a national facility for detecting fetal haemotological disorders led in 1983 to the funding of a service at King's College Hospital, London which DHSS has continued to support.

(ii) Clinical genetics

About 30 genetic or congenital disorders affect 1 in 50 children seriously enough to cause early death or lifelong disability (Tables 6.3 and 6.4). They cause 1 in 5 perinatal deaths, and over half the cases of mental handicap. Many people feel threatened by them because of family history or maternal age, often compounded by misunderstanding and misinformation. They also incur heavy costs, and their prevention offers the possibility of large savings, as well as relief of suffering.

111

Table 6.3: *Incidence and burden of common important genetic disorders in the UK. (From Weatherall[2] with additions and amendments.)*

Condition	Birth incidence per 10,000	Average years of Unimpaired life	Impaired life (& degree of impairment)	Lost life years
AUTOSOMAL DOMINANTS				
*Adult polycystic kidney disease	8	30	30(30%)	10
*Huntington's chorea†	5	40	10(50%)	20
Neurofibromatosis	4	20	30(50%)	20
*Retinoblastoma (treated)	3	3	? (20%)	?
*Myotonic dystrophy†	2	40	10(50%)	20
Tuberous sclerosis†	1	5	45(80%)	20
Multiple polyposis	1	20	30(20%)	20
AUTOSOMAL RECESSIVES				
*Cystic fibrosis	5	2	10(50%)	30
*Phenylketonuria (treated)	1	60	10(10%)	0
Neurogenic muscle atrophy	1	1	4(90%)	65
Early onset blindness	1	5	70(50%)	0
Non-specific mental retardation†[1]	5	0	50(90%)	20
*Sickle cell disease	0.5[2]	30	20(20%)	20
*Thalassaemia major	1 [2]	0	35(20%)	35
Tay-Sachs disease†	0.4[3]	0	3(90%)	67
X-LINKED RECESSIVES				
*Duchenne muscular dystrophy	2	4	16(60%)	50
*Haemophilia A	1	0	60(20%)	10
X-linked mental retardation†	10	0	50(80%)	20
CHROMOSOMAL ABNORMALITIES				
Down's syndrome†	12	0	35(80%)	35
Autosomal structural aneuploidy	5	0	20(95%)	50

Note: [1] Includes polygenic forms.
  [2] 50 per 10,000 in the ethnic groups most affected.
  [3] 4 per 10,000 in the Jewish population.
  * DNA markers available.
  † Indicates a cause of mental handicap.

Table 6.4: *Important common congenital malformations. Incidence and risk*

Condition	Incidence/ 10,000 births	%	Recurrence risk % siblings
*Anencephaly ± spina bifida†	20–300	0.2–3.0	5
Cardiac malformations	60–80	0.6–0.8	3
Spina bifida (without anencephaly)	3	0.03	5
Hydrocephaly (without spina bifida)	5–14	0.05–0.14	5
Talipes equinovarus	10	0.1	3
Cleft lip/palate	10–20	0.1–0.2	4
Cleft palate	5	0.05	2

* Not compatible with life.
† Wide geographical variation.

112

Risks are exposed by diagnosis in affected families and by screening. Genetic counselling links detection with prevention by offering guidance to individuals and their families on the possibility of developing a particular disorder or transmitting it to their children, and on ways of avoiding it or easing the consequences. Primary prevention depends on giving people reliable information on which to base decisions about having a family, and secondary prevention on influencing the outcome of a particular pregnancy by prenatal intervention.

The application of advances in molecular biology, most notably of recombinant DNA technology, has given clinical genetics fresh impetus. It has already improved the precision of detection, and exclusion, in individuals at risk of common single gene disorders. These now include adult polycystic kidney disease, Huntington's chorea, retinoblastoma, myotonic dystrophy, cystic fibrosis, sickle cell disease, thalassaemias, Duchenne muscular dystrophy and haemophilia. To these will soon be added tuberous sclerosis; and others will follow.

The refinements of prenatal diagnosis offer precise information early in pregnancy and the uncertainty which accompanies difficult decisions on parenthood is thereby reduced.

Recent advances have been made largely in disorders which are due to a single gene defect. They have a birth incidence ranging from 1 in 200 in some populations to 1 in 10,000 or less in others. There has been little impact in common disorders which result from the interplay of several genes and external factors. Among them are neoplasms, diabetes, coronary heart disease, connective tissue disorders, manic depressive illness and forms of dementia.

The concern of clinical genetics in these types of disorders will be different. Reproductive choice will not often be an issue. Risk detection will be designed to allow increasingly specific guidance to be given to individuals on preventive measures. Environmental factors such as diet, smoking and potential chemical hazards will receive attention. In some instances the non-physical environment may also be important.

The Department has funded a Special Medical Development in 3 genetics centres to determine how parents will respond to the introduction of the new genetic technique and the clinical and support activities which would follow. The results of the Development and its evaluation will be helpful to NHS planners.

In a recent joint statement[1], the Medical Royal Colleges presented brief but comprehensive views on the needs for planning and development. The statement is cognate with other documents on the provision of services published from 1978 onwards.

Effective clinical genetics is largely an out-patient specialty whose work must be co-ordinated with other specialties, especially family practice, obstetrics, paediatrics, and the investigative specialties. But genetic disorders may affect any system of the body and patients of all ages and they may be encountered in every specialty.

Wider issues
The importance of clinical genetics to medical practice, its contribution to the quality of health care and disease prevention, and the implications of recent developments for provision of services are clear[2]. There are also important social and ethical issues. The most sensitive is prenatal diagnosis and possible termination of pregnancy.

The natural means by which genetic characteristics emerge precludes the genetic make-up of an individual being known before conception. Prenatal screening and diagnosis therefore have a necessary role if reproductive decisions are always to be sufficiently informed; there is an inescapable dilemma.

The development of presymptomatic screening and diagnosis of genetic and congenital disorders arouses ethical questions of individual autonomy and informed choice, and emphasises the importance of medical confidentiality. Certain disorders are unevenly distributed between different cultural and ethnic groups and require the most thoughtful handling, as does the identification of particular families and individuals. Less sensitive, but still important, the introduction of presymptomatic screening should be preceded by careful evaluation of health benefits in the widest sense, the disadvantages and costs. The planning, organisation and delivery of services must take care to avoid predictable mishaps.

Genetic counselling
Genetic counselling provides the human link between genetics and preventive medicine. Individuals and their families who are at risk of a disorder that might be hereditary may seek advice on the possibility of developing and transmitting the disorder, of the consequences of doing so and of ways in which they may be prevented or eased. The value of counselling depends on accurate diagnosis and familiarity with the natural history of a disorder and the possibilities of intervention. It needs a keen sense of the difficulties that accompany poignant human decisions. Above all counselling needs to be sensitive to the interplay of many conflicting factors that influence choice on matters concerned with reproduction, and which heighten the dilemmas that couples face.

References

[1] Royal College of Physicians of London, Royal College of Pathologists, Royal College of Obstetrics and Gynaecologists, Royal College General Practitioners. *Need for co-ordination the development of effective genetic services (London):* Royal College of Physicians of London) 1986.
[2] Weatherall D J. The new genetics and clinical practice. 2nd ed. Oxford: Oxford University Press, 1985.

(iii) Human infertility services and embryo research

Since the Committee of Enquiry into Human Fertilisation and Embryology (the Warnock Committee) reported[1] in 1984 there have been some important scientific developments in this field in the UK and elsewhere. These include improvements in techniques for preserving embryos by freezing them for later use and the development of methods of freezing oocytes. Gamete intra-fallopian transfer has been introduced into clinical practice. This involves collecting oocytes from the ovary and, after mixing with sperm, putting them directly into the fallopian tubes. This is a valuable treatment for some couples with unexplained infertility.

Consultation on the Warnock Report in 1984 and 1985 resulted in responses which focussed on the regulation or prohibition of research involving human embryos, and on surrogate motherhood. There were relatively few comments on other important recommendations in the Report such as those about the statutory control of *in-vitro* fertilisation or donor insemination, or the legal status of children born following egg or embryo donation. Therefore in 1986 the Government, which had already indicated its intention to introduce comprehensive legislation as soon as practicable, decided that a further period of consultation was necessary before legislation could be brought in.

The Consultation Paper[2], published in December 1986, invited comments on what terms of reference and composition would be appropriate for a statutory licensing authority for certain types of infertility treatment (particularly *in-vitro* fertilisation, donor-insemination, and egg or embryo donation); whether there was a need for counselling of couples prior to these treatments to be a statutory requirement; and on ways in which a system of registering and recording children born as a result of donor insemination or egg/embryo donation might be set up. Views were sought on how best such a registration system might: (a) meet the child's need for access to the truth about his genetic origins and some information about his genetic father; (b) satisfy the family's need for privacy; and, (c) take account of the donor's wish for anonymity. Comments were also invited on the storage and disposal of embryos and inheritance; the legal status of children born as a result of donor insemination or egg/embryo donation; and on some aspects of surrogacy.

References

1. Department of Health and Social Security. *Report of the Committee of Enquiry into Human Fertilisation and Embryology*. London: HMSO, 1984 (Cmnd 9314). Chairman: Dame Mary Warnock.
2. Department of Health and Social Security. *Legislation on human infertility services and embryo research: a consultation paper*. London: HMSO, 1986 (Cmnd 46).

(i) Artificial Limb and Appliance Services

(i) The Artificial Limb Service

Preparations were well under way by the end of 1986 for the introduction of general management into the ALA Service. With the appointment of an ALAC manager in each of the 14 Health Authority regions, each centre will be able to become more responsive to the individual needs of patients. For the Artificial Limb Service this is a major advance in the manner in which health care is delivered.

(ii) Prosthetic developments

(a) — An earlier trend towards the use of energy storing/energy releasing artificial limbs has continued and several types have now been tested. A flexible below knee prosthesis was found to enhance sports performance, and two varieties of energy storing feet allowed greater recreational activity and also better negotiation of uneven terrain. These new developments are presently relatively expensive but every indication is that artificial limbs of the future will increasingly incorporate such features when the cost reduces.

(b) — A new method for above knee socket fitting (contoured adductor trochanteric controlled alignment mechanism — CAT-CAM) and similar techniques are being evaluated. For the first time the ischial tuberosity is being deliberately placed within the top of the socket and this leads to a much greater medio-lateral stability and rotational control of the prosthesis. It is expected that this concept will prove a considerable advance over more traditional methods.

(c) — A solid, silicon rubber digital or partial hand cosmetic replacement is being developed and promises to be helpful where a conventional, full prosthesis would be inappropriate. This is a welcome addition to the field of cosmetic restoration.

(iii) Wheelchairs

That the ALA Service has a responsibility for providing the necessary support systems (cushions, restraints, moulded seats etc) as well as the wheelchair itself is now acknowledged. For the first time a discrete budget for this purpose has been provided.

(iv) Birmingham symposium

The Annual DHSS/RCS Symposium took place in Birmingham on 31 October 1986.

(v) Statistics

Table 6.1 shows that in 1986 there were 5,638 new patients (254 more than in 1985). The overall ratio of arm amputations to leg amputations was 1:29.1. There were 275 non-amputation cases.

The overall ratio of male to female was 1.98:1 (1.97:1 in 1985).

116

Table 6.1: *First attendances at Artificial Limb Centres, England 1986 (Total first attendance for 1985 in parentheses)*

	Male	Female	Total	
Single arm amputations	123	57	180	(164)
Single arm non-amputations †	69	55	124	(132)
Single leg amputations	3,145	1,628	4,773	(4,450)
Single leg non-amputations †	23	18	41	(31)
*Double arm amputations	—	1	1	(5)
Double arm non-amputations †	2	1	3	(8)
**Double leg amputations	370	128	498	(494)
**Double leg non-amputations †	5	2	7	(2)
Other multiple amputations	7	—	7	(11)
Other multiple non-amputations	2	2	4	(7)
	3,746	1,892	5,638	(5,394)

† (e.g. congenital shortening, polio etc).
* Includes double arm, previously single.
** Includes double leg, previously single.

Table 6.2: *Number of first attendances for injuries resulting from Trauma, 1986 (Figures for 1985 in parentheses)*

	1986	
Trauma injuries: Total (Amp and non-amputations)	532	(484)
Arm trauma (Amp and non-amputations)	163	(145)
Leg trauma (Amp and non-amputations)	363	(335)

The male to female ratio for the 0–9, 10–59, 40–79, 60–79 and 80 and over age groups were: 1.17:1, 3.34:1, 2.28:1, 2.08:1 and 0.92:1. The corresponding ratios in 1985 were 1.28:1, 3.69:1, 2.25:1, 2.03:1 and 0.84:1.

The ratio of arm to leg amputations following trauma (Table 6.2) was 1:2.23 (1:2.3 in 1985). The corresponding ratio of arm to leg amputations due to disease was 1.98:3 (1:78.4 in 1985).

Prostheses for non-amputees
Table 6.3 lists the reasons for providing a prosthesis to non-amputees, with 76.5% of cases being congenital limb malformations.

Reasons for amputations
In 1986 a total of 3,480 (63.7%) of all leg amputations (Table 6.4) were performed for peripheral vascular disease (PVD). The figure for 1985 was 63.9%. Of all amputations 20.2% were recorded as being undertaken for diabetes mainly because of vascular complications. PVD and diabetes have accounted for 83.9% of all lower limb amputations (86.6% in 1985). This modest reduction is not considered statistically significant.

If other levels of amputation are excluded, the overall percentage of above knee amputations (including through knee procedures) to below knee amputations (including Symes) was 52.7%:47.3% (53.0%:47.0% in 1985). Despite the desirability of preserving the knee joint whenever possible there has been no discernable improvement.

Road traffic accidents (Table 6.5) — pedestrians, riders, or occupants of road vehicles — accounted for 255 attendances (i.e. amputations and non-amputations). This is an increase of 32 cases from 1985. The number of two-wheeler drivers seen has again risen this year to 127 (109 in 1985).

Table 6.3: *Reasons for providing a prosthesis to non-amputees*

	Male	Female	Total	% Total non-amputations*
Trauma	33	6	39	21.8
Congenital	61	66	127	70.9
Disease †	7	6	13	7.3

* (e.g. Patella tendon bearing (PTB) brace for non-union of tibia and fibula or flail arm splint).
† Causing shortening, instability and wasting.

Table 6.4: *Patients seen for the first time at Artificial Limb centres in England 1986 (Amputees and non-amputees)*

(i) Age distribution	Male	Female	Total	% Total
Age range				
0–9	68	58	126	2.2
10–19	90	30	120	2.1
20–39	284	80	364	6.5
40–59	694	210	904	16.0
60–79	2,186	1,053	3,239	57.5
Over 80	424	461	885	15.7
Total	3,746	1,892	5,638	100.0
(ii) Reasons for amputations				
Vascular	2,295	1,185	3,480	63.8
Metabolic				
i Diabetes	729	374	1,103	20.2
ii Other	4	5	9	0.2
Trauma	394	99	493	9.0
Malignancy	112	92	204	3.7
Neurogenic deformity				
i Acquired	15	9	24	0.4
ii Congenital	30	15	45	0.8
Infection (including gas gangrene)	66	35	101	1.9
Total	3,645	1,814	5,459	100.0

Table 6.5: *Analysis of main reasons for amputation and details of road accident cases, England 1986*

	Male	Female	Total	% Vascular cases
(a) Breakdown of vascular aetiology				
Arteriosclerosis	2,064	1,026	3,090	88.8
Embolism	130	79	209	6.0
Thromboangiitis	20	5	25	0.7
Varicose ulceration	29	32	61	1.8
Others	52	43	95	2.7
				100.0

	Male	Female	Total	% of Trauma Aetiology
(b) Breakdown of trauma aetiology				
(Amputation and non-amputation)*				
Total	427	105	532	
Industrial	91	12	103	19.4
RTA	186	26	212	39.8
Pedestrian	49	21	70	13.1
Home	23	21	44	8.3
Recreation	21	6	27	5.1
Armed forces	13	1	14	2.6
Rail	21	5	26	4.9
Other	23	13	36	6.8
				100.0

	Male	Female	Total	% of Total RTA
(c) Breakdown of RTA and Pedestrian cases				
Total	212	43	255	
Pedestrian	46	20	66	25.9
2 wheeler driver	122	5	127	49.8
2 wheeler passenger	6	3	9	3.5
Other vehicles				
Driver	27	3	30	11.8
Passenger	11	12	23	9.0
				100.0

* See footnote to Table 6.3 for explanatory example on non-amputation following road accidents.

(vi) The vehicle service

An analysis of the motor vehicles and wheelchairs on issue is shown in Table 6.6. As in recent years, the increasing number of disabled drivers opting for the cash benefit of the Mobility Allowance or the War Pension's Mobility Supplement has meant a continued decline in the powered vehicles and private care allowances on issue.

The total number of motor vehicles on issue at 31 December 1986 was 6,153 a decrease of 1,050 on 1985.

Table 6.6: *Analysis of vehicle and chairs on issue in England at 31 December 1986 (Figures for 1985 in parentheses)*

(a)	Motor cars	1,721	(2,263)
	Petrol propelled three wheelers	4,364	(4,847)
	Electrical propelled three wheelers	68	(93)
	Private car allowances (PCA's)	17	(45)
(b)	Non-powered wheelchairs (including spinal carriages, pedal and hand tricycles)	462,844	(432,013)
(c)	Powered wheelchairs		
	Indoor electric chairs	11,864	(10,548)
	Outdoor electric chairs	8,263	(7,966)
	Total	489,141	(457,775)

Table 6.7: *Patients using the Artificial Limb, Vehicle and Appliance Service in England in 1986 (Figures for 1985 in parentheses)*

Artificial Limb Service	61,770	(61,891)
Vehicle Service*	438,778	(429,663)
Appliance Service	12,867	(13,406)

* Figures in Table 6.7 refer to patients whereas Figures in Table 6.6 refer to number of vehicles on issue. A patient may have a motor vehicle or private car allowance, a powered chair and one or more wheelchairs.

(vii) The appliance service

Charged under Royal Warrant with the prescription and supply of orthoses to War Pensioners, the service is responsible for 12,867 pensions (Table 6.7), a decrease of 539 on the number for 1985.

Note: This is the last occasion on which the Artificial Limb and appliance Services will contribute to this report.

7. DENTAL HEALTH

(a) Trends

Latest figures from the 1983 and the 1985 General Household surveys (GHS) confirm the trend towards better dental health revealed by the Adult Dental Health Surveys of 1968 and 1978 and their equivalents for children of 1973 and 1983. For example, the edentulous in England and Wales has dropped from 37% of the adult population with no natural teeth in 1968, through 29% in 1978, 25% in 1983 and 22% in 1985. These figures indicate that very few people are now becoming edentulous since it must be borne in mind that as each cohort ages it carried with it those who were previously edentulous. This places limitations on the magnitude of improvement that can be attained. The extent of the fall in the edentulous population between 1978 and 1985 indicates that the rate of occurrence of total loss of teeth over this period was substantially less than in the previous 10 years. However, national statistics conceal regional and social class variation. In 1985, total tooth loss amongst adults aged over 15 years ranged for men from 12% (Greater London) to 27% (north); for women from 18% (Greater London and outer metropolitan) to 37% (north) and for men and women together from 6% (professional) to 39% (unskilled manual). The GHS of 1985 also indicates that the trends in regularity of attendance at the dentist have improved compared with earlier surveys.

(b) General Dental Services

The number of estimates authorised for payment by the Dental Estimates Board (DEB) in 1986 was 32,269,432 in England, an increase of 2.8% compared with 1985. The presentation of Dental Estimates Board (DEB) statistics changed this year. The profession and DEB agreed with the Department that in future the General Dental Service (GDS) statistics should be based, on a financial year rather than a calendar year.

Direct comparisons with 1985 are not possible but the 1986/7 data indicate some interesting trends. This information must be subject to review when next years strictly comparable data are available. It appears the number of permanent teeth filled and extracted continued to decrease, while courses of treatment involving the provision of either crowns or bridges continued to increase. For children the trend seen in 1985 toward few extractions of decidous teeth continued. The number of general anaesthetics administered also appeared to decline.

During April of this year the information given in the Department's publication *'Guidance for Surgeons, Anaesthetists and Dentists dealing with Patients Infected with HTLV III'* was distributed to all dentists employed within the NHS together with advice on cross-infection control issued in a covering letter from the Chief Dental Officer.

(c) Dental Reference Service

Dental officers in the reference service of the Department carried out 22,370 clinical examinations largely at the request of the DEB for advice on selected patients for whom treatment (excluding orthodontic treatment) was planned or had been completed. They were broadly in agreement with the plans for the treatment in 59.6% of cases. Among those patients for whom treatment had been completed they judged that it was wholly or mainly satisfactory in 95.7% of cases. The reference service also examined 1,868 patients who had received orthodontic treatment.

(d) Committee of Enquiry into unnecessary dental treatment

The Committee of Enquiry chaired by Mr. S G Schanschieff, JP, FCA published its report in February 1986. Ministers, endorsing the committee's approach, have announced that 32 out of the 52 detailed recommendations had been or were in the process of being implemented.

A further 15 recommendations were under discussion. The main areas of progress included work to develop new and enhanced systems for the DEB's new computer and to second a statistician to the DEB to assist in this respect. A review of prior approval requirements was being undertaken and the information available to patients had been revised in a leaflet and included references to the complaints procedures. The DEB also began publication of an occasional newsletter to practitioners to assist in the interpretation of the regulations. Family Practitioner Committees received advice on their role in the detection and monitoring of unnecessary dental treatment. The complement of the Dental Reference Service has been increased and a study implemented aimed to increase the effectiveness of the service.

(e) Vocational training in the General Dental Services

During the year agreement was reached with the profession to introduce a voluntary self-funding one-year vocational training scheme for graduates who wish to enter general dental practice. The Chief Dental Officer set up a committee to facilitate the introduction of the scheme which is due to come into operation on 1 January 1988. The basis of the Scheme is that graduates will be employed as assistants and work under the close supervision of experienced dentists. They will also attend on a part-time basis courses designed to give a thorough grounding of both the clinical and administrative aspects of general practice. The trainees' salaries, academic costs and trainers' allowances will be met from the Vocational Training Fund set up for this purpose. Arrangements are in hand for the selection of trainers and trainees and it is planned that each region shall have at least one scheme. It is hoped to provide places for up to half of the dental graduates entering the GDS by the year 1990.

(f) Hospital Dental Services

The total whole-time equivalent of staff in the Hospital Dental Services rose slightly from 1,192.8 in 1984 to 1,199.0 in 1986 but within this figure the numbers of staff in the specialty of Oral Surgery declined by 6.3%. The number of staff in the specialties of Orthodontics, Restorative Dentistry and Paediatric Dentistry showed an overall increase of nearly 13%.

The number of annual clinics held in all dental specialties increased from 95,521 in 1984 to 96,949 in 1985. The number of new out-patients decreased from 616,644 to 614,962; total attendances decreased from 2,743,326 to 2,701,045. The number of day cases increased from 30,849 to 33,812 and the oral surgery in-patient waiting list declined marginally from 51,797 to 51,254.

(g) Community Dental Services

The maintained school population in England on 1 January 1985 was 7.43 million. This represents a decrease of just over 4% from the 1983 figures. The percentage of the school population inspected had increased to 71% although the number of school children inspected had decreased marginally. Just over 5.2 million children were inspected in schools or clinics and of these 35% required treatment, a decline of 7% in the number requiring treatment recorded in 1983.

Between 1983 and 1985 the number of handicapped adults inspected rose by more than 72% to 50,559. The number of handicapped adults treated rose by over 66% to 30,055 but the proportion inspected who were treated declined from 62% to just over 59%.

The whole-time equivalent of all staff employed in the community dental service declined from 1,416.8 in 1984 to 1,405.0 in 1986. However, within this figure the numbers of senior dental officers increased by over 12% to 279.2 and the number of dental officers decreased by nearly 5% to 967.3.

(h) Dental manpower

The Departmental Study Group Report on Dental Manpower was published in 1983. The background leading to the initiation of the study was included in *this Report* for that year (page 86). The Report advised that systematic and periodic review of dental manpower would be necessary and recommended, among other things, that the next review should be set up when the GHS 1983 data were available. This survey was published in 1985 and included information on trends in total tooth loss and also in dental attendance patterns.

The discussion document on Primary Health Care published in April 1986 announced that a further review would be undertaken. Discussions with the British Dental Association (BDA) began in the summer of 1986 with consideration of a paper produced by the BDA on future dental manpower needs.

The aims of the review were to decide whether the trends forecast in the 1983 report still held good and whether or not the respective weighting attached to those trends should be altered, with particular emphasis on revised estimates on future levels of demand and supply. For the first time, the review group has examined the geographical distribution of dentists as it is quite clear that the availability of general dental practitioners around the country varies a great deal. The group's report will be completed by the middle of 1987, after which the precise methods of achieving a balance between demand and supply will be the subject of negotiations between the Department and wider professional interests.

(i) Primary health care

The Agenda for a discussion document published in April 1986 was the subject of a full consultation process which ended on 31 December 1986. Among the dental subjects about which the Government sought to promote discussion was an increased emphasis on the role of prevention of dental disease. The

Government had asked health authorities in areas where dental health is poor or the level of attendance at the dentist is significantly below the national average to consider the benefits of water fluoridation schemes with particular care. Following the publication in 1985 of the report of the Director General of Fair Trading which looked at the availability of the NHS treatment the Government welcomed the relaxation by the GDC of restrictions of advertising by dentists. However, the discussion document explained what further changes could be made to improve consumer choice and service availability of NHS dentistry for the public. Also explored were the changes in the contract of employment for dentists which might be beneficial. These included the question of a retirement age for dentists and the range of NHS treatment which was available.

As described elsewhere in this chapter the improvements to training made possible by the Vocational Training Scheme for general dental practice were explored and a scheme introduced. In conjunction with professional and academic interests other issues considered in the field of education and training included the need for post-qualification refresher training in the context of the likely future changes in clinical techniques and materials.

The place of the Community Dental Service was considered and suggestions were discussed for a change of role for the service with development towards greater emphasis on dental health education, group prevention programmes, screening in areas of special need, and the treatment of people who for other reasons, require special consideration including handicapped groups.

(j) The safety of dental amalgam

The Committee on Toxicity completed a comprehensive review of the scientific evidence of the safety of dental amalgam and advised as follows:

"Dental amalgams containing mercury have been used for 150 years and we understand that in the United Kingdom some 30 million amalgam restorations are inserted each year. Despite this extensive usage only a very few cases that can be recognised as having a reaction to mercury occur each year, and these are due to hypersensitivity. Nevertheless, from time-to-time concern is expressed in some quarters that use of dental amalgam may lead to excessive exposure to mercury and to poisoning.

We have examined the evidence from which such concern arises. There is some evidence that mercury is released from dental amalgam during the period following insertion and on the removal or restorations. Some mercury may be released as a result of corrosion but this is likely to be small because of the excess of unreacted alloy in the finished filling. The development of copper enriched alloys has reduced the potential for corrosion. Vaporisation of mercury from amalgam restorations may possibly occur with prolonged heavy chewing. However, long term clinical evidence would seem to suggest to that substantial amounts of mercury are not released from amalgam fillings.

Theoretical considerations suggest that in extreme cases the amount of mercury released might, were it known to be absorbed, constitute an undesirable although not a toxic exposure. However, studies of the concentration of mercury in the blood of people with amalgam restorations indicate to us that the exposure is in fact of no toxicological significance. It has been suggested also that exposure to mercury from amalgam may be a factor in the development of some chronic diseases, but in out opinion the evidence does not support his contention.

In our opinion the use of dental amalgam is free from risk of systemic toxicity and only a very few cases of hypersensitivity occur. It is our view that further research in this area would not merit priority''.

This advice was subsequently endorsed by the Committee on Dental and Surgical Materials.

8. NHS ORGANISATION AND MANAGEMENT

(a) The Regional review process

Regional Performance Reviews were introduced in 1986. They complement the existing annual cycle of Ministerial Reviews in which ministers hold Regional Health Authorities (RHAs) to account for their stewardship of health service resources. In Ministerial Reviews ministers meet Regional Chairmen, but Performance Reviews are meetings between members of the NHS Management Board and officers of the RHA.

The Chief Medical Officer is a member of the NHS Management Board. His attendance ensures that a range of relevant medical items are at these meetings. In the first cycle of reviews particular emphasis was placed upon health promotion, immunisation and vaccination, and cervical screening services. It is intended that progress in these areas will be discussed in the next cycle, and additional topics will be introduced.

(b) Non-clinical support for hospital medical and dental staff

The provision of secretarial support for hospital medical and dental staff has been the subject of debate for some years. Changes in the organisation and delivery of clinical services, new management arrangements and the advent of modern information technology have all created pressure for change. With the help of the Joint Consultants Committee (JCC) a working party was set up in 1985 to examine these issues. It was asked to make recommendations about the recruitment, organisation and management of the non-clinical support staff, including medical secretaries, who are required by hospital medical and dental staff to enable them to deliver a safe and effective service to patients. The Working Party was asked to take into account the resources likely to be available.

The Working Party has completed its report, and the report has both been commended by the JCC and accepted by the NHS Management Board. It was issued to health authorities on 23 January 1987.

(c) Hospital complaints procedure

Current arrangements for dealing with complaints from hospital patients are based on a memorandum of guidance [HC(81)5] which was circulated to health authorities in April 1981. The memorandum referred to the handling of complaints of a non-clinical nature and to a separate, but linked, procedure for investigating complaints involving the clinical judgement of hospital medical or dental staff. The latter is a three stage procedure agreed with the JCC, which may involve two independent consultants, nominated by the JCC, reviewing the case and reporting their findings to the Regional Medical Officer.

A Private Members Bill led to the Hospital Complaints Procedure Act (1985). The intention of the Act is that the current permissive guidance relating to hospital complaints procedures will be replaced by statutory directions. Consequently wide consultations on revised complaints procedures were undertaken during the year with a view to improving current procedures and issuing directions to health authorities during 1987.

(d) Relations with the MRC

(i) Concordat
The arrangements for co-operation between the Health Departments and the MRC agreed in the Concordat in 1980 were reviewed in 1986. They were found by both sides to have been largely satisfactory. The new document differs from its predecessor only in points of detail:

(1) the arrangements for the annual 'stocktaking' meeting are more flexible;

(2) MRC's commitment to expenditure on health services research is updated to £2.8m per annum at 1986 prices and Council have undertaken to endeavour to expand the health services base within their own research structure; and

(3) there is more flexibility in the Health departments' representation at MRC Board meetings.

(ii) HSR Committee
In 1980, following Council's endorsement of the Concordat, the MRC established a Health Services Research (HSR) Panel to advise on applications in the field. However the Panel became increasingly concerned at its inability actively to encourage HSR and in 1984 it reported to Council that it should have an executive function with authority to award grants and to promote the development of HSR. In 1985 Council agreed to reconstitute the Panel as the Health Services Research Committee with a limited executive function for an experimental period of 3 years.

The Committee's terms of reference are:

(1) To foster high quality HSR (in collaboration with the Health departments, and with the ESRC as appropriate) in areas of interest to the MRC;

(2) To advise Council and Boards on policy relating to HSR and on any matters that are referred to the Committee;

(3) To assess project and special project grant applications in the field of HSR and make awards up to the limits of the Committee's budget; and to advise the appropriate Board or Council or other applications for grants and on proposals arising from Council units or Institutes;

(4) To consider how the problems of training in HSR might be solved; and to advise the Training and Manpower Committee accordingly; and

(5) To assess reports of MRC work with significant HSR content.

The Health Departments have welcomed the steps being taken to encourage submission of HSR grant applications to the MRC and also the increased emphasis for training in HSR.

(e) National external quality assessment schemes for pathology laboratories

These Schemes provide an important mechanism whereby the standard of performance pathology laboratories in the UK is maintained. Schemes are funded by the DHSS in all the pathology specialties but any action which is required to draw the attention of participating laboratories deficiencies in their performance, and to assist such laboratories in improving their performance, is taken by the relevant professional bodies. The Schemes are open to all laboratories, both NHS and private, and further efforts were made during 1986 to ensure that more private laboratories participated. These efforts are still continuing and most private laboratories now participate in relevant Schemes.

During 1986 work continued to expand the range of assays covered by the Schemes and new Schemes for HIV antibody analysis and for parasitology were introduced. Preliminary work was carried out to enable a pilot Scheme for the monitoring of urine drugs of abuse assays to begin in 1987.

For the first time an Annual Report covering the activities of all the Schemes was published. This was widely distributed to Regional and District administrators, professional bodies and overseas. The Report was well received and will be produced annually in future.

(f) Safety of medical devices and equipment

The objective of DHSS policy on medical equipment procurement is to assist the NHS in purchasing at an economic price, products fit for their intended purpose, particularly with regard to safety and quality in order to protect users and patients. One corner-stone of safety is the compliance with a relevant Standard (British or International). Another is the non-statutory control scheme run by Procurement Directorate which has 3 main features: (i) registering manufacturers who have good process and quality assurance and withholding registration from those who do not; (ii) user assessment reports from experts in NHS centres; and (iii) the reporting of defects and problems encountered in practical use.

To assist the monitoring of newer implanted devices, 2 databanks have been established. The one for pacemakers at the National Heart Hospital contains information on about 55,000 pacemakers, of which 37,000 are active as implants. During 1986 there were about 10,200 new implants in the UK, nearly 80% of which were captured in this scheme. This databank ensures the immediacy of the Department's defect investigations.

The second databank is that on cardiac valve replacement, established in January 1986 and mentioned in *this Report* for 1985 (p. 78). This has now completed its first formal year of data collection. A preliminary report has been prepared which will enable us to look back on what has been achieved and also review methods of data collection and analysis.

(g) ACARD report

The Government's response to the ACARD report was published in February 1987. It welcomed the report and accepted that the NHS has an important part to play as the major purchaser of medical equipment in the UK. NHS decision makers should be aware of both their influence on the shape of the UK medical equipment industry and the need for value for money within the health service. The establishment of the NHS Procurement Directorate in January 1986 with the Supply Technology Division as an integral part is a welcome development. The functions of the Procurement Directorate relate directly to patient care. The Director of NHS Procurement has addressed the JCC and has established ongoing liaison with Royal Colleges, professional bodies and the NHS.

A new option appraisal manual for medical supplies and equipment has been prepared and a draft is out for consultation with the NHS. It will give those responsible for the NHS purchasing decisions guidance on how financial resources should be used. Priorities in Health Technology Assessment are being addressed by the newly formed DHSS Chief Scientist's Health Technology Assessment Group.

A new Medical Equipment Research and Development Co-ordinating Group has also been formed which includes representatives from DHSS, the Department of Trade and Industry, the Science & Engineering Research Council and the MRC. This will explore ways of implementing the co-ordination of the sponsorship of Medical Equipment Research and Development.

(h) Computing within the NHS and the National Strategic Framework

The increasing importance and usage of information technology in the Health Service is well recognised by the Department. The national strategic framework for information management in the hospital and community health services was issued in October by the Information Management Group to Health Authorities and relevant professional bodies. The basic principle contained in the document states that information technology is a valuable resource which is provided and used by all levels of the health service and as such should be managed well. Regarding the usage of information technology generally within the NHS, the recommendations from Körner reports are being implemented in stages by Health Authorities and this is proceeding well.

(i) Family Practitioner Committee (FPC) computers
There has been progress in the installation of FPC computers. The programmes included on the computers include patient registration and the cervical cytology 'call and recall' modules. It is hoped that all systems will be in place by the target date of March 1988.

(i) Planning, manpower, medical education

Effective planning and control of medical manpower is essential for the successful provision of health care. During 1986 there have been two major initiatives which seek to make an improvement in the structure of hospital medical staffing and one which has focussed on long-term planning.

In July 1986, a consultative document *'Hospital Medical Staffing: Achieving a Balance'* was published[1], following discussions between the medical profession, the Health Departments and RHA Chairmen. If implemented, the recommendations will bring about the most significant changes in the medical staffing structure in hospitals for many years. The aim is to correct the present imbalance between the number of consultant posts and the number of junior doctors training for them particularly registrars. Correction of this imbalance by increasing the proportion of clinical work carried out by consultants and by improving the morale of the juniors will contribute to improved patient care. The report recommends several measures to increase the number of consultant posts, a reduction in the number of registrars, the introduction of a new intermediate level service grade and improved methods of relating the number of UK doctors in training to career opportunities. It also makes recommendations which will facilitate early and partial retirement for consultants and which will improve training for junior staff. A Steering Group under the chairmanship of the Minister for Health is now meeting to consider comments made during the consultative phase and to oversee implementation. A pump-priming scheme to fund 100 additional consultant posts over the next two years in General Medicine, General Surgery and Traumatic and Orthopaedic Surgery was announced in February 1987.

A Joint Planning and Advisory Committee (JPAC) has been considering, within the medical specialties, the number of senior registrar posts required to fill expected consultant vacancies. Within the last year scrutinies have been carried out on 11 specialties; a further 17 are planned for 1987 and the rest will be conducted in 1988. Each specialty will then be kept under review. For the specialties already scrutinised JPAC has set manpower targets to be achieved within the next 5 years. This will lead to an increase in some specialties and a decrease in others, and like the changes mentioned above will improve the balance between the numbers of career posts and trainees in hospitals.

Emphasis has also been placed on long-term planning and a second Advisory Committee for Medical Manpower Planning (ACMMP II) was set up in April 1986 to look at likely trends in manpower supply and demand well beyond the ten-year horizon of Health Authorities' strategic plans. The Committee comprises nominees of the medical profession, the Universities, the Health Service and Health Departments.

In the broad area of education the training, the Department is financially supporting 3 of the Royal Colleges (Physicians, Surgeons, and Obstetricians and Gynaecologists) to develop educational sponsorship schemes for overseas doctors coming to the UK for postgraduate training in hospitals. Doctors wishing to benefit from these schemes will need to achieve a high academic standard before arriving here and appointments will be to substantive training posts (at senior house officer and registrar levels mainly) in specialties relevant to the needs of their home country.

Their training and performance will be closely monitored. The eventual aim is that most overseas doctors wishing to train in the UK will come under a recognised sponsorship scheme. The Department has also given evidence to the Croham Committee which reviewed the funding of medical education through the University Grants Committee. The Croham Report makes clear recommendations on the need to co-ordinate planning and funding activities on the health and education sides and on the need for close liaison between the DES and the Health Departments[2].

References

[1] Department of Health and Social Security Joint Consultants Committee. Hospital medical staffing: achieving a balance: a consultative document issued on behalf of the UK Health Depart-

ments, the Joint Consultants Committee and Chairmen of Regional Health Authorities. Department of Health and Social Security, 1986.

² Committee on the Review of the University Grants Committee. *Review of the University Grants Committee: report of a committee under the chairmanship of Lord Croham, GCB*. London: HMSO, 1987: 50–5 (Cmnd 81).

(j) Waiting lists

In September 1986, 681,901 people were waiting for in-patient treatment in NHS hospitals. Since the health service began this number has been around 500,000. It started to grow during the 1970s broadly in line with the increase in acute sector activity. Despite the bigger lists, the time that patients had to wait for admission remained the same from 1975 to 1985, averaging 7 weeks. Hidden within this average are wide variations and in some areas and in some specialties too many patients wait too long. One-quarter of the patients on the non-urgent waiting list in September 1986 had been there for over a year, and three-fifths of those on the urgent list had been waiting for over a month. This was a major national problem in terms of the quality of service provided by the NHS.

In July 1986 a 3-year initiative was announced to shorten waiting lists and waiting times. The Secretary of State asked RHAs to report on the nature, extent and cause of problems in every district. These reports showed that significant improvements were already planned or being made within existing resources in many districts but that more could be achieved with extra money. In November 1986, the Secretary of State established a waiting list fund of £50m spread over 2 years to support projects aimed at making improvements in problem areas.

DHAs and RHAs submitted bids for projects to be supported from the fund in 1987/88, and these were scrutinised by Sir Roy Griffiths, Deputy Chairman of the NHS Management Board. In February 1987, the first £25m was allocated to fund over 350 projects for treating more than 100,000 extra in-patients nationwide. Included in this total will be 5,000 hip replacements and 8,000 cataract operations as well as extra day care work. This will be achieved by re-programming the use of facilities, extending working hours in the evening and at week-ends, and purchasing minor pieces of equipment. The private sector and spare capacity in neighbouring health districts may also be used.

RHAs have been asked to monitor progress closely both on the schemes supported by the waiting list fund and on other actions within existing resources to improve waiting lists and times. The introduction of the Körner data system will make such supervision easier in years to come but during the first year of operation some problems in data capture and disjunction in time sequence comparisons are inevitable.

The waiting list is a complex phenomenon and attempts to reduce waiting times have implications strategically for levels of acute activity as compared with services for priority groups, and managerially for working relationships between clinicians and managers. The aim of the project team under the direction of Sir Roy Griffiths is to develop and to promulgate a better understanding of factors that lead to excessive waiting lists and waiting times and so improve the targetting of further stages in the initiative.

9. SOCIAL SECURITY

(a) Industrial injuries

The Social Security Act 1986 introduced a number of changes to the Industrial Injuries Scheme. While some of these will not apply until 1987, the following ones began during 1986.

Disablement assessed at less than 14% in respect of claims made after 30 September 1986, other than those for exempt diseases (pneumoconiosis, byssinosis and diffuse mesothelioma) does not attract Disablement Benefit. Disablement assessed at 14% or more attracts payment of a disablement pension and where the assessment lies between 14% and 19% this payment is at the level appropriate for 20%. For an award of Disablement pension, the Adjudication Officer may aggregate disablement arising from a claim after 30 September 1986 with that from an earlier or later claim. The effect of this will be that, even if an individual claim will not in itself attract benefit, taken in conjunction with assessments for earlier or later claims it may do so. Claims made before 1 October 1986 remain subject to old rules, up to and including any final assessment.

Special Hardship Allowance is abolished, to be replaced by Reduced Earning Allowance. This is no longer an increase of Disablement Benefit, but is a separate benefit. The underlying condition for an award is either payment of Disablement Benefit or continued relevant disablement of at least 1% (20% in the case of occupational deafness).

These changes in the law required further alterations in the boarding forms, in addition to those referred to in *this Report* for 1985 (p. 101). However, these alterations were not as extensive, though the commencing date of 1 October 1986 required their implementation to be accomplished more quickly. This has meant that 2 fundamental changes in procedure have had to be put into effect within a period of a few months. It was not possible, in the time available, to launch a pilot scheme, but comprehensive guidance notes were issued to all members of Medical Panels, and guidance sessions were conducted by Departmental medical and non-medical staff as appropriate.

Two new occupational respiratory diseases were prescribed with effect from 1 April 1985. These were primary carcinoma of the lung where there was accompanying evidence of either asbestosis or bilateral pleural thickening, and bilateral diffuse pleural thickening; 34 cases of the former and 11 of the latter condition were diagnosed in 1986. The figure relating to lung cancer is an under-estimate as the condition complicating previously diagnosed asbestosis was treated as being due to the asbestosis since this procedure was more advantageous to the claimant.

In occupational asthma 7 more subjects were added to the list of agents prescribed with effect from 1 December 1986. The new agents are antibiotics, cimetidine, wood dusts, ispaghula powder, castor bean dust, ipecacuanha and azodicarbonamide.

(b) Severe disablement allowance (SDA)

Two changes occurred towards the end of 1985 which affected the processing of claims to SDA at medical adjudication sections in 1986. First, from 25 September 1985 the practice of referring all cases to a medical officer to consider whether the necessary level of disablement could be accepted on the basis of documentary evidence (paper boarding) was abandoned and all but a number of selected cases were referred directly for medical examination. Secondly, people aged 35–39 years became eligible for benefit from 28 November 1985 resulting in a large increase in the numbers of cases being referred for examination.

Since the introduction of SDA, claimants who were registered blind or partially sighted in England and Wales automatically received SDA without having to undergo examination to assess their disablement (passporting). Because registration in Scotland does not require the opinion of an ophthalmologist, blind claimants from Scotland had to undergo examination before they could receive SDA. From 8 December 1986 passporting arrangements were extended to include blind and partially sighted claimants from Scotland.

(c) Attendance allowance

Attendance allowance, the first non-contributory disability benefit, was introduced in 1969, the first payment being made in 1970. In the original concept it was to be a non-contributory, non-means tested cash benefit paid to the long-term disabled to enable them to employ help to look after their bodily functions, or to supervise them if this was required to avoid danger to themselves or others.

The benefit was originally paid on a one-tier basis, those fulfilling the medical criteria day and night from 2 years of age onwards received the payments weekly for a period specified by the adjudicating authority. Based on a survey carried out in the period 1960–65 the number of beneficiaries was estimated at 25–30,000, 40,000 at the outside.

During 1972 it became obvious that the numbers had been grossly under-estimated. The benefit was extended in 1973 and the payments divided into day and night, creating a lower and higher rate. At that time there were 152,159 benefits in payment, 107,534 at the lower and 44,625 at the higher rate. The changes were incorported in the 1975 Social Security Act and various key elements (night and day, bodily functions, attention/supervision, the meaning of 'frequent' substantial danger) were defined either by decisions of the Social Security Commissioners or the High Court (mainly Lord Widgery and Lord Denning).

Perhaps as a result of increased publicity from these judgements or the formation of various groups dedicated to helping people with particular disabilities, claims increased dramatically during the years 1980–1985. In the same period the machinery built up by the DHSS also matured and it is now possible to clear an uncomplicated claim in 6.5 weeks (from the time the claim is handed in to the claimant receiving the first payment). Although there is scope to reduce this even further, there is an absolute limit made up from postal delays and the sheer physical time a file movement takes. Considering the numbers involved, it is not overlong, even though this will not help the occasional delayed claim.

(d) War pensions

In 1986 war pensions attracted much publicity. The Department published a new leaflet (FB16) which explained briefly who was entitled to a war pension and how to claim. The leaflet was distributed to ex-service organisations, local DHSS offices, War Pensions Welfare Offices and Local Health Authorities. At the same time articles in the press and on television drew the public's attention to war pensions. As a result of all this there was a significant increase in war pension claims at the end of 1986 which has spread through into 1987.

(e) Mobility allowance

The numbers of claims for this benefit have increased every year over the last 5 years and so have the number of beneficiaries. This increase has resulted in extra workloads at all levels but improvements in efficiency have reduced the average processing time from approximately 14 weeks in 1982 to just over 7 weeks in 1986.

(f) Statistics

	1985	1986
Industrial injuries		
Disablement benefit claims (excluding prescribed respiratory disease)	197,640	211,263
Prescribed respiratory disease		
New claims	8,192	7,547
Total — all claims	24,603	22,895
Occupational asthma cases agent		
Isocyanates	46	48
Platinum salts	9	12
Hardening agents	19	28
Soldering flux	25	20
Proteolytic enzymes	6	0
Animal/Insects	7	12
Flour/Grain	54	46
Severe disablement allowance		
Paper boards	7,728	3,040
Medical examinations	11,631	23,333
Appeals to MAT	802	2,132
Number in receipt of benefit	251,900	263,000
Attendance allowance		
Claims	277,000	287,000
Total allowances in payment		
Higher rate	222,000	237,000
Lower rate	321,000	348,000
Total	543,000	585,000

		1985		1986
Mobility allowance				
Number of beneficiaries		400,211		454,644

War pensions

		1986		
Monthly new claims	January	555	July	686
	February	669	August	737
	March	578	September	837
	April	591	October	821
	May	733	November	741
	June	523	December	1,230

10. INTERNATIONAL HEALTH

(a) The World Health Assembly

The 39th World Health Assembly was held in Geneva from 5 to 16 May 1986. The UK delegation which was led by the Secretary of State for Social Services included Dr I S MacDonald, CMO of the Scottish Home and Health Department. He contributed to the technical discussion on the role of inter-sectorial co-operation in national strategies for Health for All.

The Assembly reviewed the first worldwide evaluation of the strategy for achieving Health for All by the year 2000.

The exercise revealed encouraging trends such as a greater resolve to improve people's health, better statistics for immunisation procedures and for maternal and child health, improvements in the standards of drinking water and a continuing rise in life expectancy at birth (60 years or more in 96 countries). Unfortunately, the overall situation still gave cause for deep concern.

Infant mortality rates are 100 per 100,000 births or more in 44 countries representing 30% of the world's population. Health infrastructures are still weak in most countries with formidable problems in ensuring that the essential elements of primary health care are provided. Lifestyles in developed countries are leading to more illness from cardiovascular diseases and from cancer and this pattern is beginning to show up in the developing countries. Ageing of the population places heavier burdens on the Health and Social Services and urbanisation is taking place before plans for the prevention of its adverse consequences have been implemented.

The UK delegation contributed to the discussions on a wide range of subjects. The Chief Nursing Officer emphasised the key role of nurses in health care systems and argued for nurse education to move away from the medical model. She recommended that the input of the nursing profession to national health strategy planning should increase. Members of the delegation supported the demand for stronger action against smoking and spoke about AIDS, the rational use of drugs, psychotropic substances, and nutrition of infants and young children. The UK was a member of a working group set up to re-draft a resolution calling, amongst other things, for the cessation of the supply to maternity wards of free or subsidised supplies of breast-milk substitutes. The resolution was approved by the Assembly by 92 votes to 1, with 6 abstentions, but a number of delegations reserved their positions on this operative paragraph pending further consideration of the matter with the competent authorities of their own countries.

The Health Assembly also decided to re-assign Morocco, at its request, from the European Region to the Eastern Mediterranean Region; to increase membership of the WHO Executive Board from 31 to 32; and to change the name of the Advisory Committee on Medical Research to the Advisory Committee on Health Research.

(b) WHO Regional Committee for Europe

The 36th Regional Committee took place in Copenhagen from 15 to 20 September 1986. Sir Donald Acheson was elected Chairman.

Table 10.1: *Age standardised mortality rates per 100,000 population (males and females) — Age-group 0–64 years (except for RTA's and Suicides)*

	Diseases of the circulatory system	Ischaemic heart disease	Cerebro-vascular diseases	Malignant neoplasms all causes	Lung cancer	Cancer of the cervix	RTAs all ages	Suicides all ages	(Crude death rates) Infant mortality rate per 1,000 live births	Maternal mortality per 1,000 live births
England & Wales (1984)	108.92	79.46	16.86	100.68	25.58	5.00	9.26	8.47	9.48	0.08
France (1984)	54.19	21.35	13.28	99.50	17.47	2.14	29.15	21.30	8.29	0.14
Federal Republic of Germany (1985)	82.6	44.70	13.45	88.82	17.21	3.34	11.79	18.63	8.95	0.11
Netherlands (1984)	76.44	48.13	11.17	89.85	23.83	2.67	10.64	12.52	8.36	0.10
Denmark (1984)	85.22	58.81	12.17	104.00	26.49	5.95	12.18	28.19	7.66	0.08
Greece (1984)	65.92	31.24	17.37	75.10	18.22	1.55	20.57	3.84	14.34	0.09
Luxembourg (1985)	91.24	45.04	21.50	104.58	22.98	1.81	21.17	14.27	8.28	0.00
Norway (1984)	82.27	58.61	11.45	74.80	12.94	3.56	9.82	14.52	8.33	0.02
Sweden (1985)	73.73	50.83	10.47	69.78	10.90	2.43	9.23	17.22	6.75	0.05
Finland (1984)	120.78	82.73	20.00	74.07	18.26	1.35	10.27	24.75	6.62	0.02
Italy (1981)	78.55	34.98	19.01	96.33	22.19	1.01	17.46	6.71	14.13	0.13
Ireland (1983)	127.05	89.25	19.41	97.66	23.54	3.10	15.52	9.25	10.13	0.12
Belgium (1984)	82.04	39.49	13.99	98.33	26.17	2.82	18.72	22.65	9.77	0.09
Spain (1980)	74.29	25.20	19.38	76.17	12.08	1.30	16.76	4.69	12.41	0.11
Portugal (1985)	76.13	24.86	31.24	78.07	10.00	2.24	25.47	9.86	17.83	0.10

Data supplied by the WHO European Regional Office

Table 10.2: *WHO and Council of Europe medical fellowships administered in the UK during 1986*

	WHO Fellowships commenced in UK during 1986							Average duration in months	Council of Europe fellowships commenced in 1986	Total fellowships commencing in 1986
	Europe	Eastern Mediterranean	Africa	South East Asia	West Pacific	Americas	Total			
Public health and administration	5	19	16	6	11	2	59	5.5	5	64
Environmental health	12	7	3	3	—	2	27	2.5	1	28
Nursing	3	10	7	2	5	7	34	6	6	40
Maternal and child health	6	1	5	3	—	2	17	6.5	3	20
Communicable diseases	8	8	2	7	2	1	28	3	1	29
Clinical medicine	12	26	7	9	3	6	63	6	16	79
Basic sciences	10	7	10	10	10	5	52	7	4	56
Other health services	5	11	10	16	17	—	59	4	5	64
Total	61	89	60	56	48	25	339	5	41	380
Average duration in months	2	6	11	4.5	3.5	4				

WHO Fellowships Programmes requested during 1986 but cancelled   53

WHO Fellowship Programmes already in progress at 1.1.86   175

Other Programmes arranged during 1986   11

The Committee reviewed the European region's proposed programme budget for 1988–89, which had been re-structured to bring it into line with the presentation of the European Regional targets. Proposals for the region's programme of work in the biennium were endorsed.

The Committee chose the European region's campaign against tobacco as the theme of its first concerted action. Multi-sectional national programmes to contain the AIDS epidemic in Europe were also approved.

(e) Commonwealth Health Ministries meeting

The eighth Commonwealth Health Ministries meeting took place in Nassau from 13 to 17 October. The British delegation was led by Lord Glenarthur, Minister of State at the Scottish Office and the Departmental team was led by Dr E L Harris, Deputy Chief Medical Officer.

The British delegation took part in all 3 Committees covering specific aspects of health financing. There was general agreement that a tax-based system of health financing was the most efficient form of funding. Such a system would help to ensure equity in health care delivery. The importance of sound financial and manpower planning was stressed. Governments were urged to consider how better use could be made of non-governmental organisations and the extent to which private sector health care might contribute to health care delivery. The need for more bilateral health assistance to be concentrated in key areas was also discussed. The meeting stressed the importance of better co-ordination between Ministries of Health and Donor Development Agencies.

(d) International mortality rates

In 1984 Member States of the European Region agreed a set of targets to support European strategies to implement Health for All by the year 2000. The WHO Regional Office for Europe has supplied the latest information about 6 of the outcome targets (and their related sub-targets) which relates to mortality rates in the EC and Scandinavia. (Table 10.1). The data update similar age standardised mortality rates published in *this Report* for 1984 (p 112).

(e) Who and Council Europe Medical Fellowships

During 1986 the Department was involved in 567 programmes for WHO Fellows visiting the United Kingdom: 339 of them started their programmes which lasted on average for 5 months. Fifty-three programmes were initiated but cancelled either by WHO or the Department before studies began and 175 were in progress on 1 January 1986. Towards the end of the year the Department began discussions with the European Regional Office of WHO on setting up a computerised data-base of training facilities for WHO Fellows in the European Region.

Forty-one Council of Europe Medical Fellows came to the United Kingdom for periods ranging from 15 to 60 days. Eleven programmes were arranged for visiting officers from international or national Health Administrations. Details are shown in Table 10.2.

WHO awarded 6 and the Council of Europe 7 fellowships for studies overseas during 1987 to UK candidates. The periods of study will range from 1 week to 3 weeks.

APPENDIX A

(i) Members of the Committee on Safety of Medicines

Professor Sir Abraham Goldberg MD DSc FRCP FRSE (Chairman)
Regius Professor of the Practice of Medicine, University of Glasgow

Professor A W Asscher MA BSc FRCP
Professor of Renal Medicine, University of Wales, College of Medicine,
Royal Infirmary, Cardiff

Professor M Breckenridge MD MSc FRCP
Professor of Clinical Pharmacology, Liverpool University

Dr C M Castleden M D FRCP
Consultant Geriatrician, Leicester General Hospital

M W Darling Esq OBE FPS
Chairman South Tyneside Health Authority

Professor J W Dundee MD PhD FRCP FFA RCS
Professor of Anaesthetics, Queens University, Belfast

Professor P H Elworthy BPharm PhD DSc MSc CChem MRSC FPS MCPP
Emeritus Professor of Pharmacy, University of Manchester,
Visiting Professor of Pharmaceutics King's College and the School of Pharmacy,
University of London

Professor A T Florence DSc PhD FRSC MPS MCPP
Professor of Pharmaceutics, University of Strathclyde

Professor D G Grahame-Smith MB BS PhD FRCP
Rhodes Professor of Clinical Pharmacology, Radcliffe Infirmary, Oxford

Professor M W Greaves MD PhD FRCP
Professor of Clinical Dermatology, St Johns Hospital for Diseases of the Skin,
London

Dr J M Holt MA MSc MD FRCP
Consultant Physician, John Radcliffe Hospital, Oxford

Professor D Hull BSc FRCP DObst RCOG DCH
Professor of Child Health, University Hospital and Medical School, Nottingham

Professor H S Jacobs BA MD FRCP
Professor of Reproductive Endocrinology, The Middlesex Hospital Medical
School

Dr B L Pentecost MD FRCP
Consultant Physician, Birmingham

Professor M D Rawlins BSc MD FRCP
Professor of Clinical Pharmacology, University of Newcastle-upon-Tyne

Dr J W G Smith MD FRCPath FFCM FIBiol Dip Bact
Director, Public Health Laboratory Service Board, London

Professor M P Vessey MB MD FFCM
Professor of Social and Community Medicine, Radcliffe Infirmary, Oxford

Dr D M B Ward MB ChB
General Practitioner, Glasgow

Professor K H Weinbren BSc MD FRCPath
Professor of Experimental Pathology, Royal Postgraduate Medical School, Hammersmith Hospital

Note
Term of office for all members expired 31 December 1986.

Members Appointed for Specific Meetings

January	Professor M J S Langman BSc MD MBBS FRCP
	Dr A V P Mackay PhD MA BSc MRCP
	Dr G Schild BSc PhD FIBiol
February	Dr A V P Mackay PhD MA BSc MRCP
March	Professor D W Mathieson PhD BSc CChem FRSC
	Dr D P Thomas DPhil MD FRCPath
May	Professor M Elstein MD FRCOG
	Dr J L Mann DM PhD
July	Professor A McMichael PhD CMAA MRCP
	Dr G Schild BSc PhD FIBiol
	Dr A E Theobald BPharm PhD MPS
	Professor E S Williams MD PhD FRCP FRCR
September	Professor B Bridges
	Professor M H Lessof MA MD MB BChir FRCP
	Professor A E M McLean BM PhD FRCPath
December	Professor D W Mathieson PhD BSc CChem FRSC

(ii) Members of Sub-Committees (CSM, CRM and CDSM)

Sub-Committee on Safety, Efficiency and Adverse Reactions
Professor D G Grahame-Smith MB BS PhD FRCP (Chairman)
Professor A M Barrett BPharm PhD
Professor A M Breckenridge MSc MD FRCP
Dr D M Davies MD FRCP
Professor M Elstein MD FRCOG
Professor A M Geddes MD FRCP
Dr W A Jerrett MB BCh FRCGP
Professor D H Lawson MD FRCP (Ed)
Dr A V P Mackay BSc MA PhD FRCPsych
Professor J O'D McGee MD PhD FRCPath MA

142

Professor A E M McLean BM PhD FRCPath
Professor M D Rawlins BSc MD FRCP
Professor R I Smith PhD DSc
Professor J F Smyth MA MSc MD FRCP
Dr I Sutherland DPhil
Professor J D Swales MA MD FRCP
Dr P J Toghill MD FRCP DObst RCOG
Professor H K Weinbren BSc MD FRCPath
Professor V Wright MD FRCP

Sub-Committee on Chemistry, Pharmacy and Standards
Professor P H Elworthy BPharm PhD DSc MSc CChem MRSC (Chairman)
Dr M L Alwood BPharm PhD MPS
Professor B W Barry BSc PhD MPS CChem FRIC
Professor J R Brown BSc MSc PhD MPS CChem FRSC MIBiol
Dr D H Calam MA DPhil CChem FRSC
Dr R T Calvert BSc PhD MPS
Professor J E Carless Pharm MSc PhD FPS
Dr F Fish BPharm PhD FPS
Professor A T Florence BSc PhD CChem FRSC MPS (Vice Chairman)
Dr B P Jackson BPharm BSc PhD FPS FLS
Professor D W Mathieson BSc PhD CChem FRSC
Dr E B Mullock PhD MRSC CChem
Professor J M Newton BPharm PhD FPS
Dr J D Phillipson MSc DSc PhD FPS FLS
Professor A Tallentire MSc PhD FPS
Dr D Watt PhD MSc FPS

Sub-Committee on Biologicals
Dr J W G Smith MD FRCPath FFCM FIBiol Dip Bact (Chairman)
Professor J E Banatvala MA MD FRCPath DPH DCH
Professor W J Brammar BSc PhD
Professor J G Collee MD FRCP FRCPath
Professor G C Jenkins MB BSc PhD FRCPath
Professor H Keen MD FRCP
Dr R S Lane MD MRCP MRCPath
Professor A MacMichael PhD CMAA MRCP
Professor J Melling BSc MSc PhD FIBiol FPS
Professor E R Moxon MB BChir FRCP
Dr D P Thomas DPhil MD FRCPath
Dr D A J Tyrrell CBE MD DSc FRCP FRCPath FRS
Mr J G Watt BVMS MRCVS

*Joint CSM/JCVI Sub-Committee on Adverse Reactions to Vaccines and
Immunological Products*
Professor R W Gilliat DM FRCP (Chairman)
Dr Sir John Badenoch DM FRCP
Professor J E Banatvala MA MD FRCPath DPH DCH
Dr A L Bussey MB BS FFCM DObstRCOG AMBIM
Dr P E Fine VMD PhD
Professor A A Glynn MD FRCP FRCPath
Professor D Hull BSc FRCP DObst RCOG DCH
Professor J K Lloyd MD FRCP DPH

Dr B W McGuinness MD FRCGP DObstRCOG DCH RCPS
Dr C L Miller BN BCh
Professor D L Miller MA FRCP FFCM DPH MD
Dr J W G Smith MD FRCPath FFCM FIBiol Dip Bact
Dr D Reid MD FFCM DPH
Dr S J Wallace FRCP DObst RCOG

Printed in the United Kingdom for Her Majesty's Stationery Office
Dd.289942   C18   GP443   11/87   4073